EYE

ON

LEADERSHIP

STEVE VARGO, OD, MBA

Steve Vargo, OD, MBA

Optometric Practice Management Consultant

IDOC

© 2017 by Dr. Steve Vargo

Contents

Introduction

"Alone we can do so little. Together we can do so much."
— Helen Keller

How do I motivate employees?

That's a question I am asked frequently. It probably won't surprise you to hear that there's not a simple answer. But on the bright side, the process is not incredibly complicated either.

Let's look at the above question a little closer. What are you really asking?

> How do I get employees to work harder or faster?
> How do I get employees to go the extra mile?
> How do I get employees to do what I ask?
> How do I get employees to **CARE**?

The topic of motivation and teamwork often fails to acknowledge leadership's role in cultivating a motivated and collaborative work environment. "It's hard to find good people" is a complaint I hear often, but an organization that lacks effective leadership will often struggle to get the maximum production out of ANY of its employees. When I analyze the top producing practices I have consulted with, I routinely observe a more proactive approach to leadership and a commitment to shaping the office culture to fit the leader's vision. These efforts result in a more engaged and committed staff, allowing the doctor to spend more time on growing the practice and less time dealing with staff-related problems and drama.

But I'm not good at managing people!

While I do think that some people have stronger leadership skills than others, I have also observed people in leadership positions use the "I'm not good at managing people" mantra as an excuse for neglecting staff management responsibilities. The good news is that everything I mention in this book is very practical and actionable. The topic of leadership can become very esoteric and philosophical. This book is about the fundamentals. If you are in a leadership position and have ever thought or said "I'm not good at managing people", I had you in mind when I wrote this.

Let me add that I do not think there is one right leadership or management style. Professional sports serve as a great example, as some of the most successful coaches are known for being very quiet and analytical, whereas others are very vocal and demanding. This is a personal preference shaped by your own personality. You have to do you. This book is not intended to shape your individual leadership style as a business owner; it's meant to give you the foundational building blocks to be a more effective leader. Anyone can do this, regardless of your comfort level or abilities with managing other people.

Why is leadership important?

I'm paying my employees! Why can't I just tell people what to do and expect them to give me their best effort? That's a fair question, but your rationale here will lose out to the science of human behavior. As a rule, money tends to be a poor motivator. You have to look deeper if you want to understand what motivates people. Leadership is not about imposing your will on others, it has more to do with understanding people. A draconian, micromanaged work environment tends to keep people in compliance but often fails to inspire employee engagement and commitment. In the right environment, even average employees will volunteer their best (or at least better) effort. Decades of science and research have revealed a wealth of information on how to motivate people, yet business owners and people in leadership positions continue to ignore these principles. Fighting the basic tenets of human behavior is a losing battle.

And let's not overlook this very important point. In an industry that is increasingly impacted by disruptive technology like online refraction sites and Internet vendors, the service component is becoming the major differentiator for brick and mortar businesses. The service your team provides is a direct reflection of the culture that leadership instills. Neglect that, and you leave yourself severely exposed to outside threats.

5 habits of effective leaders

In 2014 I transitioned from clinical practice to full-time practice management consultant. About one year into my new role a client asked me a very pointed question. "How do I motivate people?" I realized at that moment that I really didn't have a good answer. I had worked with numerous practices on issues related to underperforming employees, but I didn't have a clear, coherent answer for this OD. So I set out to find one.

I began by reviewing past consults with consulting clients pertaining to underperforming employees. Having done hundreds of consultations with doctors all over the country on staff management issues alone, I began to identify **5 key areas** that I focused on about 90% of the time when discussing an underperforming employee. While I was happy to have a "framework" for motivating employees, I then quietly asked myself, "Am I giving *good* advice?"

That question took me outside the optometry profession. I looked at companies outside our industry known for creating high-performing teams that consistently delivered great performance. What were they doing to motivate and engage employees? I was happy to learn that my advice was very closely aligned with the tactics and strategies used by these companies. I feel very confident that the five principles presented in this book can be leveraged by any practice to significantly improve staff performance and office culture.

These are not necessarily revolutionary ideas; in fact most of these are time-tested management principles taught in business schools and implemented by many of today's top companies. However, as with many business strategies, execution is where many leaders stumble.

> "My staff won't do it."
> "My employees don't like change."
> "They did it for a few weeks and then went back to doing it the old way."
> "They're just not motivated!"

This book provides the information, but execution is up to you. My goal is to provide insight along with actionable ideas for motivating your team that can easily be implemented into any optometry practice. If you are stuck on the proverbial hamster wheel of managing a practice, it's time to consider a new approach. Some small but powerful changes can dramatically improve your staff performance and office culture. The challenge is to incorporate these ideas into your skill set and do them consistently - every day. In the book *Good to Great: Why Some Companies Make the Leap... And Others Don't*, author Jim Collins identified disciplined people doing disciplined things every day as one of the hallmarks of companies that went from Good to Great!

It starts with you!

This book was written in story format. It's the story of 3 individuals in different stages of their business life—an optometrist, a local business owner, and a business consultant. It's a journey of sorts as this unlikely trio meets once a month at an Irish pub to discuss business and life, and how the two intertwine. Although the characters and story are fictitious, it mirrors many of the challenges I hear daily pertaining to staff management. The goal of this book is not to make you a better boss; the goal is to make you a better leader. It starts with you, and you are the main character in this story.

Now take the field. It's game time!

Chapter One:
An Intriguing Offer

"If you want to go fast, go alone.
If you want to go far, you need a team."
— Coach John Wooden

"One or two?"

"Excuse me?" you ask the young man who just singled up the middle knocking in two runs.

"How many outs are there, one or two?"

"Oh. There's one out." Your reply sounds more like a question than an answer. Coaching your son's baseball team has been a great distraction from all the problems going on in your eye care practice. However, lately the stress has been mounting. Even concentrating on your coaching duties has been a challenge. You remind yourself to pay attention to what's happening on the field, but your mind is never far away from all the challenges you are experiencing as owner of an optometry practice.

Since you opened your practice cold three years ago, several new practices have opened in your town. You didn't anticipate this level of competition. You also didn't anticipate the challenges this would create around staffing. In the past year three of your best employees left to work for a competitor. They cited better pay as the reason, but it also came to your attention that these employees were generally unhappy working at your practice. The people you hired to replace them have been mediocre employees at best. You are constantly fixing their mistakes and putting out the daily fires that pop up, not to mention the never ending drama that a few of your employees are fond of creating. Motivation? At this point you've all but given up on expecting your employees to deliver high-level performance. You just wish they would do the job they've been hired to do. It feels like most of the time they are doing just enough work to not get fired. Revenues and growth in the practice have been stagnant, and while you have ideas to turn that around you lack the time to implement these ideas. You spend most of your time in a dark room doing eye exams, with most of your discretionary time spent firefighting and trying to keep your head above water. Even if you had the time, you suspect that the staff would be an obstacle to implementing these ideas. Your attempts at introducing improvements in the past were met with resistance and excuses.

When you opened the practice there were only two employees, and the other was your wife Katie. Even though money was tight, these were exciting times! The practice was growing. You and Katie made a great team! You shared a unified vision around creating the kind of practice that you both wanted. Patients liked your practice and you were growing through word of mouth. But that was then, and this is now. As the practice grew and you began adding new employees, the culture deteriorated. Some "bad apples" hijacked your vision and replaced it with their own agenda. By the time you recognized the problem, several negative reviews and increased staff turnover had made a strong impact on the practice. The local competition became a more attractive option for many of your patients, and word of mouth was no longer driving new patients into your practice, it was driving people away. Katie had to get another job to help pay the bills and only occasionally helps out at the practice. It's no longer just the business debt that is mounting; it's also personal debt. Financial troubles combined with disagreements over how to manage and operate the practice have led to problems at home. Some days you stay late at the office even when there are no patients to avoid another argument with Katie. Most days you feel alone and defeated. Whatever vision you once had as a business owner, this wasn't it.

As you ponder your situation from the first base coach's box, your son Lucas rounds first base after hitting a line drive into left field. He looks up and asks, "How many outs dad?" You have no idea.

A burger and a beer

"I wish managing employees was as easy as coaching these kids." Unaware anyone was listening as you mumbled those words under your breath, a voice behind you says, "What do you mean by that?" The unexpected reply came from Tim Hughes. Tim is the head coach of the Acworth Warriors, the baseball team you both coach.

"Oh, sorry," you blurt out, "I'm just having some problems with my employees. I wish they would listen as well as these kids do," you say as you're pointing toward the field.

"What do you do for a living, Kevin?" Tim asks.

"I'm an optometrist," you respond.

"Ah, a doctor! Then I should call you Dr. Kevin," Tim half-jokingly offers.

"Nah, Kevin is ok with me. Besides, I'm not feeling like a very good doctor these days."

"Oh? Why is that?"

"Well, it's not so much the doctor part I'm struggling with, it's the business part. Apparently I'm not very good at managing people, or maybe I'm not good at hiring people. Either way, I feel like I'm on an island by myself trying to run a business. Some days I wonder if it's even worth it." You decide to cut yourself off here, fearing Tim was just looking for friendly chitchat.

Tim, however, finds this very interesting. In fact, he finds this surprising. You see, in the six years that Tim has coached his son's Little League teams, he has found you to be one of the best assistant coaches he has worked with. There is an art to coaching kids at sports and not everybody gets that. Aside from the occasional zoning out while coaching first, you are very good with the kids. They like playing for you and the parents pick up on that. You make it fun and they show up eager to learn. Most the parents have seen dramatic improvements in their kid's abilities, even the ones that lack a great deal of athletic prowess. You also have a lot of patience with the kids and see most situations on the field as opportunities to teach. You raise your voice when the situation calls for it, but in order to make improvements the kids need to understand when they have done something wrong that needs correction. Your greatest joy as a coach is seeing kids improve as the season progresses. The kids love playing for Coach Kevin. Tim wonders to himself why you are so good at managing little leaguers but struggle to successfully manage your employees.

"Kevin, what are you doing after the game today?" Tim asks.

"Hmm. Well, I was crossing my fingers for another romantic evening at home arguing over bills with the wife," you laugh awkwardly.

"Tell you what, drop Lucas off at home and meet up with me for a burger and a beer. I'm meeting a friend at O'Donovan's Pub. I think you'll enjoy meeting him."

You accept the invitation, not quite sure what to expect, but at this moment preferring a burger and a cold beer to another argument at home.

Table for three

The establishment chosen for this meet-up has some history for you. This is where you and your wife originally hatched the idea to open up your own practice. You were working for a local chain optical and regretting the time you had to spend away from your family working evenings and weekends.

It was only temporary you kept telling yourself, but the years kept ticking away. You saw your kid's ball games through the verbal accounts they provided when you got home from work. Aside from some weekend getaways with the family, you had not taken Katie on a vacation since your honeymoon. She occasionally hinted about vacationing in the Caribbean, but realizes that will likely not happen anytime soon. Even if you had more time away from work, money was also an issue as you struggled to keep up with personal bills and student loan debt. Finally, it was time to make the move! You and your wife held up two wine glasses and cheered to the future. That feels like a lifetime ago.

As you walk in the restaurant you spot Tim and another gentleman seated in a booth near the back. Tim spots you and waves you over. As you walk up to the booth the other gentleman stands up and offers a hearty "Hello Kevin! My name is Robert Childress. Tim here was just telling me a little bit about you."

"Hi Robert," you respond while extending a handshake. "It's a pleasure to meet you."

After some small talk about local politics, sports and what burger to order, Robert breaks the ice by asking you about your job. "So Tim says you're having some problems managing the people who work for you. If you don't mind my asking, what kind of problems are you having?"

Before you can respond, Tim chimes in with an explanation that explains why he invited you out this evening. "Kevin, I should explain that Robert is a business consultant, not just a nosy friend of mine. He has helped me out a great deal in my business and I thought he might be able to help you as well."

"A business consultant?" you inquire. "What type of businesses do you consult for?"

"Well, I've worked in several industries but mostly technology firms," Robert replies.

"Oh," you say, "I'm afraid my background is in healthcare. Optometry to be specific."

"Oh, well that's a shame! In that case I guess we'll just eat our burgers and talk about something else," Robert says with a straight face. After a moment of awkward silence, Robert lets out a chuckle and says, "Look, people are people regardless of what industry you are in, and if you want to get your business right, you have to get your people right!"

This struck you as common sense, but yet sounded so intuitive when you heard someone else say it. Robert was right! You recalled the comment you made to Tim about feeling like you were alone on an island. The truth is you were not alone; you were with a tribe of villagers standing around watching you drown offshore. You needed help!

As the evening wore on, talking with Robert and Tim you become more and more convinced of your shortcomings with managing your employees and the impact this was having on your practice. As the check came, Robert made an intriguing offer. "Kevin, I'll make you a deal. Tim and I get together here once a month for lunch. If you are interested in joining us, I'm happy to share with you what I have learned over the years about managing and leading people. When you break it down to the fundamentals, it's not quite as complicated as you might think. In fact, when I look back at all the cases I've had with clients involving managing employees, 90 percent of the time I am focusing my recommendations in five specific areas. If you care to learn how to apply these principles to your eye care practice, meet up with us the next five months. That is, if you don't mind picking up the check," Robert says with a smile.

You look over at the table where you and Katie cheered to the future three years earlier. For the first time in a long time, the weight on your shoulders feels a little less heavy as a hint of optimism seeps in. "Robert," you say with an extended hand, "lunch is on me!"

Chapter Two:
Are We Clear?

"Lack of direction, not lack of time, is the
problem. We all have twenty-four hour days."
— Zig Ziglar

"Where is the next patient?" you ask a passing optician as you peek your head out the exam room door. "Kim is pretesting her," she responds. Ah, Kim - the tech who takes twice as long as every other tech to work up a patient. You would tell her to hurry up, but that hasn't worked well in the past.

As you're heading out to meet Robert and Tim for lunch, you overhear your optician open with "Let's see what your insurance covers." No surprise this is your lowest producing optician. Tami, your lead optician always discusses premium options and multiple pairs with every patient. "Why can't all my opticians go the extra mile like Tami?"

Revenues are down again this quarter. You would love to have more time to focus on growing the practice but you are constantly putting out fires related to staffing issues. "Isn't this why I hired an office manager?" you grumble as you overhear two staff members arguing over who is responsible for doing patient recall. Your manager's response to these staffing issues is usually to get frustrated and do their work for them. She is fond of pointing out that the employees have worked here for a while, they should know what to do! Lately she has been preoccupied with handling the billing. Accounts receivable has never been higher. You hired a billing person, but she makes a lot of mistakes.

Looking a bit frazzled from this morning's events, you meet Robert and Tim at O'Donovans. "You look a little stressed out today buddy," Tim observes.

"Ugh," you reply. "Another crazy day dealing with my staff. It's like nobody has any idea what they are supposed to be doing or how to do it!"

"What's your training process look like, Kevin?" asks Robert.

"Well, my wife handled the training when we were starting out. But as I mentioned, she has another job so now we have an office manager who handles this. The only problem is she can be very impatient and I think the staff is intimidated of her. She gets busy with her own tasks and I think she delegates some of the training to other employees. I'm afraid we don't have a good system for training. I'm also afraid a lot of bad habits get passed down during the training process."

"Do you have any process for meeting with the staff to review their responsibilities, answer questions, etc.?" Robert asks.

"Yeah, that," you ponder. "I know we should meet more but we all get busy with our own stuff and staff meetings have become a thing of the past."

"What about regular one-on-one meetings with employees?" Robert pushes.

"Well, if we're not having staff meetings, I think you probably know the answer to that one."

Robert smiles at that remark, but then unexpectedly changes the subject. "Tim was telling me your kid is a pretty good ball player," Robert says.

"Yeah," you proudly reply. "He was struggling last year but we've worked out a lot of the issues he was having."

"Tell me more about that," Robert says.

"Well, he's always been a good fielder but last year he was struggling at the plate. It got to the point he didn't even enjoy playing. I noticed his approach at the plate had changed and he had developed some bad habits. He was opening up his shoulders too early in the swing causing him to hit a lot of popups and lazy ground balls."

"How did you correct that?" asks Robert.

"We spent some time at the batting cages and put in extra work during practices. Once we identified the problem I videotaped his swing so he could understand exactly what he was doing wrong. We also watched a lot of YouTube videos showing the correct mechanics of a swing and we worked together to emulate that style. Eventually the bad habits ceased and his hitting improved."

"That's interesting," Robert remarks. "Tell me a little more about how you handle other kids who are performing below expectations."

You sense this line of questioning is going somewhere, but you're not quite sure where. "With the other kids it's a similar approach. It's the coaches job to explain to them what they are doing right and what needs improvement. It's not just their performance on the field, but it's also their knowledge of the game. They need to know where they need to be and how they need to respond in different situations. They need to know what the coaches expect in terms of attitude and hard work. They can't be expected to play their best if they are not clear on what is expected of them."

With this last remark, Robert offered a wide grin. "Kudos to you Doctor Kevin! You just discovered lesson number one!"

Lesson #1:
Be clear with expectations

As optometrists, nobody delivers clarity better than we do – literally and figuratively. Our professional lives are spent helping people see better. We also provide very clear instructions to patients to avoid confusion.

> *"This is the medication I want you to take. I want you to put 1 drop in your left eye four times a day for ten days. When you instill the drop, tilt your head back and press your thumb and index in the bridge of your nose for 10 seconds. I would like you to return in one week so I can reevaluate the condition of your eye."*

While ODs give very clear guidance and direction to their patients, as employers do you provide this same level of clarity around employee performance expectations? You may be thinking, "Of course I do. I train them after all, and we have a training manual *somewhere* around here." But ask yourself the following questions:

- Do employees ever fail to complete important tasks?
- Do they take too long to do the tasks they are assigned?
- Do they make recurrent mistakes?

- Do they ever argue over who is responsible for certain job duties?

- Do they ever spend excessive time on the wrong activities?

I've heard these very complaints from numerous employers. While it's possible this is an employee problem, it's also possible that the employee is simply unclear on his or her job expectations.

Research from Gallup discovered that 50% of employees lack clarity on what is expected of them at work. The authors of the study believe that when employees do not have a clear understanding of what's required of them, they are less engaged with their jobs. Sure, your technician knows how to perform non-contact tonometry and your billing person knows how to submit an insurance claim, but what about the technician that takes twice as long as the other techs to pre-test a patient and a billing person who makes an unacceptable number of billing errors? Before concluding that you made a poor hire, ask the following question, "Does the employee *know* he or she is underperforming?"

Consistent with the Gallup survey, approximately half the time I hear from an OD or office manager complaining of an underperforming employee, I discover that the employee has not been given adequate feedback pertaining to specific goals and expectations. Employees need to know when they are performing well and when they are not. To facilitate that, employees need clear direction on what is expected of them, how much and when. That can mean clarity of the overall direction and goals of the practice, but it could also be simple things like clarity around daily activities. Expecting your employees to always know what is expected of them will likely leave you disappointed.

Now let's focus!

Clarity and focus are often used synonymously, but they are not exactly the same. You can be clear on a lot of different priorities, but lack the focus to do any of them well or see them through to completion. By definition, not everything is a priority.

An attendee at one of our national conferences told me that he just loves coming to our events. He and his staff leave the meetings energized with many new ideas to implement into the practice. He then informed me that his staff struggles to create lasting change. After a few weeks, the staff loses momentum and goes back to doing things the "old way". In other words, they lose focus.

Time is a scarce resource in many practices. A typical day in an optometry practice involves a flurry of activity and a variety of demands competing for everyone's attention. Much of the day is spent responding to urgent, but not always important issues. Combine this with the limited time, resources and people available in most small to mid-size business. When you attempt to introduce a lot of new ideas and change into the mix, common pushback from staff is that there is not enough time. In a busy practice, they may be right!

The solution is to prioritize goals and focus on the most important. That's not to say you neglect less important areas, but you significantly increase your chances of accomplishing a task or goal when you invest more of your time, energy and resources into fewer projects. Even if you are good at multi-tasking and taking on several projects at once, most people are more productive when they can focus their time and energy on fewer priorities. There's a good chance the aforementioned practice did not abandon their ideas due to lack of motivation, but rather a lack of prioritization.

Speaking of priorities

The same Gallup study mentioned above found that employees who were **clear on work priorities** were almost **10 times** more likely to be engaged in the workplace. Engaged employees are those willing to go the extra mile, work with passion and feel a strong connection to the vision and values of the practice. They routinely deliver better

Steve Vargo, OD, MBA

service and out-produce their actively disengaged counter-parts. These are the employees who will move the practice forward.

If you desire a more "motivated" team and work environment, start by clarifying expectations and priorities for the staff. While some employees are naturally driven and self-motivated, others rely on clear direction and feedback to succeed. What appears a lack of motivation or resistance to change is often a lack of clarity.

Is this my fault?

Returning to work after the lunch meeting, you had a fresh perspective on the situation. All along you had operated under the assumption that good people were simply hard to find. Some employees were just lazy and entitled. That afternoon you watched a tech take 25 minutes to pretest a patient (15 minutes of that time was spent talking about their pets), an optician talk a patient out of getting sunglasses from your practice (according to the optician she just needs a cheap over-the-counter pair) and your front desk person make a snide remark to a patient that it's his job to understand his insurance. "Could this be my fault?" you pondered for the first time. We haven't had a staff meeting to review office procedures and expectations in almost a year, and other than an annual review that is now handled by your less than competent office manager, there's really no process for communicating performance expectations to staff. Could it be that they really don't know *specifically* what is expected of them?

Next Steps:

In the book *Why Employees Don't Do What They're Supposed To Do and What To Do About It,* author Ferdinand Fournies concludes through his research that **setting clear expectations is often a supervisor's first failure**. Managers think they have clearly stated work objectives, requirements and deadlines, but the employee received a different message. Based on responses from interviews with nearly 25,000 managers, below are the top 3 reasons stated for why employees do not do what they are supposed to do:

1. They don't know why they should do it

2. They don't know how to do it

3. They don't know what they are supposed to do

Employees who are not clear on what they are supposed to do cannot do their job very well. As a boss and leader, it's your job to get everyone on the same page. Establish specific roles and responsibilities with employees so everyone is crystal clear about expectations and can work together cooperatively. This may initially require you to write down specific roles and responsibilities, but once you've done that it's time to meet with the employees, both as a group and individually if necessary, and **BE CLEAR WITH EXPECTATIONS**!

Chapter Three:
The Smartest Guy in the Room

"Don't tell people how to do things, tell them what to do and let them surprise you with their results."

– George S. Patton

"So, Doctor Kevin, tell us about this past month," Robert eagerly requests as you assume your seat at the same booth.

Energized from last month's meeting, you begin to tell both Robert and Tim how you made a long list of all the things you wanted your staff to do and exactly how you wanted them to do it. You then closed the office for half a day to inform staff of all the mandatory changes moving forward.

You then paused for their response. The one you got you were not expecting. After a brief moment of silence, Robert and Tim looked at each other and started laughing. "How'd that go for ya buddy?" Tim asks with a smile on his face as he reached for a menu.

"Well, I'm not sure yet. They didn't really say much. I have to say they didn't look too happy about some of the things I was saying. I may be wrong, but I get the general feeling that some of them are upset with me." Robert and Tim laugh again.

"Ok, jokes over," you respond. "I just did what you suggested. What's so funny?"

"Look Kevin, I said it's important to set clear expectations for your employees. They need to be crystal clear on what is expected of them if you expect them to do their job correctly. But I never said you should micromanage your employees or dictate their jobs to them."

Tim held up a finger at this point to intervene. "Kevin, let me tell you about my own experience with this. I own Tim's Sporting Goods."

"Wait, you're *that* Tim?" you surprisingly respond.

"Yes, I'm *that* Tim, and there were numerous times in the past when I wished I was not *that* Tim. I started the business back in 2008. We had one location on the north side of town. There wasn't much competition at that time and business was good. The hardest transition for me was when we expanded and added a second location. The part I struggled with was not being able to oversee everything. And by oversee, I mean control. I had three managers for the various departments in the one location and we held weekly manager meetings. My managers hated these meetings, but I felt they were important. The meetings mostly consisted of me telling the managers what I wanted them to do and how I wanted it done. I was the one doing most the talking. I was the smartest guy in the room, or so I thought. If things were not getting done the way I had insisted, I made sure they knew about it. This was my version of managing expectations."

"I'm a little confused," you reply. "Isn't this what setting expectations is all about?"

"Technically, maybe," Tim says, "but let me tell you how my approach was very limiting when it came to getting employees to give their best efforts. As time went on, the business grew and I was no longer able to attend every manager meeting. This is about the time I started working with Robert. I explained my predicament to Robert and he asked me about my managers. Could I trust them? Are they committed to their jobs? I said yes, for the most part they were. So Robert's suggestion was for me to focus on other areas of the business that needed my attention but still insist that the managers continue to meet once a week without me. At the time I recall thinking this would be a waste of their time, but something really special began to happen when I was no longer at these meetings. They started coming up with their own ideas. And these ideas were good. These were ideas I had never considered. These ideas solved problems I was not even aware of. My perspectives were limited to what I knew, which I came to realize was not nearly adequate to make all these decisions by myself. My managers were in the trenches so to speak. They were regularly hearing from the other employees and getting feedback from the customers. Through this process I learned one of the most valuable things I have done as a business owner is to get out of the way and let my employees start making some of their own decisions."

"Wow. I've never looked at it that way but I guess that makes sense," you say. "Come to think if it, I wouldn't want to work for a boss who dictated my job to me and didn't value my input. I've had jobs like that. It wasn't a very good work environment. Nobody seemed very energized or motivated. A lot of the employees quietly disagreed with the manager's ideas to improve the workplace but since our ideas were never solicited, we didn't feel comfortable giving our input."

"Exactly!" Tim responds. "Don't get me wrong, you can't just turn over the entire operation to your employees, but if you don't involve your staff in decisions about the business then you will have a hard time keeping good people."

"But!" you interject. Tim knew a "but" was coming. "I can't allow the staff to do things I don't' agree with! I have to make a lot of decisions as a business owner and not everyone can have their way."

Tim smiled in agreement. "You're absolutely right Kevin. The employees cannot always have their way, but let me offer two thoughts on that. You're right, you are the owner and CEO of your practice and you have to make a lot of high-level decisions, but don't you think you'll make better decisions when you have more information? You see, that was my problem; by discouraging employee input and involvement I was making decisions based on limited knowledge. When things didn't go right I blamed the employees. I later realized this wasn't a problem of execution; it was a problem of strategizing. I was making a lot of poor decisions. This isn't to say that every decision I make as a business owner is a home run, but a team approach to decision making has led to a much more productive work environment and successful business."

"You said there were two things," you remind Tim.

"Oh yeah," Tim recalls. "Kevin, just because you don't agree with your team doesn't mean you are right. Take a chance on your staff from time to time. I'm not talking about anything so grand that you will lose the practice if they're wrong, but most decisions are not of that magnitude. Hire good people and roll the dice on them every once in a while. I do that frequently with my team. I tell them Ok, we'll try it your way and review the outcome at a future meeting. If it's a home run we keep doing it. If it's a dismal failure we stop doing it. What usually happens is that we learn from trying something new. We learn what works and what doesn't work and we pivot."

"Pivot?" you ask.

"Yes, pivot," Tim continues. "That means we make adjustments to fix or eliminate what's not working while capturing and repeating what is working. Pivoting is a process of continual improvement. In fact, that has become the motto for Tim's Sporting Goods – Make it Better! Perfection is never the goal; rather we strive for continuous improvement. All our decisions are based around whether they "make it better". Does it solve a problem? Does it improve customer service? Does it improve efficiency? To answer these questions, you need the full involvement of your team, not just one owner like me whose ego kept getting in the way."

"So I guess you wouldn't endorse the comment I made to my wife last night," you say as the waitress arrives with everyone's food.

"What's that?" Tim asks.

"I told her I wish I could just tell people what to do and have them do it."

Robert, not having said much to this point but enjoying Tim's story, looked up to the ceiling as he appeared to mull over your comment and then waived a French fry at you as he said "Ya know, if that's the culture you want you can be assured you will eventually get it. You'll find yourself surrounded by a group of people standing around waiting to be told what to do."

"Ok," you reply while reaching for your turkey club. "That's enough making me feel stupid for today. Let's eat."

Tim and Robert share their third laugh.

Lesson #2:
Empower your employees

In chapter 2 we discussed the importance of setting clear expectations around desired outcomes. These outcomes could include practice goals such as optical capture rate and number of patients seen as well as individual outcomes such as average time to check-in a patient or policies around tardiness. Studies in employee behavior have shown that setting clear expectations with employees may be one of the most valuable things a leader can do. Approximately half the time I consult with practices on underperforming employees, I learn that the employee has been given very limited feedback (if any) on their performance and job expectations. If feedback has been given, it's often vague and ambiguous.

While clarity of expectations is an important element of leading your team, nowhere in lesson 1 did I suggest micromanaging employees or dictating their jobs to them. I believe it's important for leaders to have a vision for the business and clearly articulate that vision to the team along with clear expectations, but I believe it's equally important to allow your staff some autonomy and independence in how these goals are reached.

Empowerment is not enough

For starters, you need a commitment from your employees that they want more authority and decision making power. While some people thrive in an autonomous work environment where they are allowed greater freedom and independence in the way they do their job, others rely on more direction and control from management. Recruitment and hiring are not the focus of this book, but if you find yourself surrounded by more followers than doers (and wished it was opposite), it may be time to analyze your hiring process. Ask job candidates to tell you about times at previous jobs where they took the lead on a task or project that added value to the organization. If you get a deer in the headlights look with that question, it's possible that either they have never been asked to contribute at this level or they've never shown the initiative.

Autonomy in the workplace has to be earned and not every employee will rise to the occasion. Some people just want to show up, follow directions and then go home. Not everybody is a go-getter, but in my personal experience and my experience working with other practices, most offices have at least a few employees who would give you greater commitment and energy if given the opportunity. I've been pulled aside at conferences by managers and staff members mentioning that they love some of the practice building ideas they heard at the conference and they have several of their own ideas that would benefit the practice, but the doctor won't support their efforts. That's a real shame! Standing before me is someone who wants to make a positive impact in the practice, and the owner is the one standing in the way! In a tone of frustration, a few have also mentioned that they are considering other employment options if things don't change. There's no better way to demotivate a motivated employee than to put him or her in a rigid environment that discourages creativity and independence.

For those who struggle with relinquishing control, understand that empowering employees is simply an act of giving them a voice. You are allowing people closest to the information to make decisions, contrary to the standard habit of pushing information to those with the authority to make decisions. As owner and CEO of your business, many of the high-level decisions still have to go through you. That being the case, you will likely make better decisions if you have good information from the people around you. Great leaders are always collecting information. Your employees are on the front lines and can provide you with information you were unaware of or solutions to problems you had not considered. Use specific words to identify the level of empowerment you want, such as "explore options," "recommend alternatives," or "come up with a plan." As Steve Jobs once said, for an organization to be successful the best ideas have to win, not hierarchy! And from a motivational standpoint, employees will likely bring more energy to their work when they are allowed to contribute to the process. People like to see their own ideas succeed!

Still not convinced?

Google did a rigorous analysis to reveal what makes a team effective. Their research concluded that even an average group of employees could perform at a high level if certain factors are in place. According to their research involving 200+ employee interviews and looking at more that 250+ attributes of 180+ active teams, the most important attribute was what they termed "psychological safety". A psychologically safe work environment is a workplace where ideas, input and suggestions are welcome without fear of ridicule or belittlement by management. Teamwork is more valued than hierarchy. Healthy debate among team members was encouraged, not punished. Input from all staff members is valued, not ignored. In this type of work environment, you will frequently find less turnover, higher morale and employees that produce at higher levels. Click HERE to read more about the study.

I can't allow that!

A consulting client once responded to the idea of empowering your team by saying "I can't allow my staff to do things I don't agree with". He made a good point. Yes, as a business owner high-level decisions have to go through you. This may apply to office managers as well. But let's consider a few things.

1. Because you do have to make a lot of business decisions, it only benefits you to have as much information as possible to help you make the best decisions. You can't say "yes" to every idea an employee brings forward, but a culture that discourages employee involvement in decisions will eventually become a culture where employees stop coming to you with ideas.

2. Just because you do not agree with your staff does not mean you are right. Take a chance on your team every now and then. If they have an idea that they think will add value to the practice or solve a problem, let them try it. Tell them you will reconvene with them at a specified date to evaluate if the idea has been a whopping success, dismal failure, or more likely some elements of both. The last scenario is actually a success. Many successful practices achieve success through some trial and error and calculated risk

taking. Through this process you learn what strategies work and which ones don't. The strategies that work ultimately become 'best practices' that you repeat.

In the previous chapter I referenced the extensive research from the book *Why Employees Don't Do What They're Supposed To Do and What To Do About It* by Ferdinand Fournies. In that chapter I listed the top 3 reasons employees do not do what they are supposed to do. Below I included the fourth and fifth reason.

1. They don't know why they should do it
2. They don't know how to do it
3. They don't know what they are supposed to do
4. They think your way will not work
5. They think their way is better

Next steps:

Strive for an inclusive, team-oriented workplace where employee's ideas and input are encouraged and valued. If your office culture has been a "top-down" approach to management where leaders make all the decision with limited or no involvement from non-managerial employees, it may take some time for employees to feel comfortable getting involved. If you just want robots to show up to work and do what they're told, this isn't necessary, but I suspect some of the people you've hired have some good ideas that they've been hesitant to suggest. Start asking for their ideas and including them in decisions. Learn to do more listening and ask more questions. Many 'lone wolf' business owners have a lot of blind spots about the operations of their business. Ultimately, you'll make better business decisions when you allow the people around you to fill in those blind spots! The previous chapter focused on providing clarity for employees, but leaders need clarity as well. Staff meetings and one-on-ones are good opportunities to have these discussions. To avoid these meetings becoming gripe sessions, give your staff permission to come to you with problems but make it a requirement that they also have proposed solutions. Try to keep these discussions focused on solutions. Remember that complaining or 'venting' is often a reactionary response to situations where we feel we have little control or involvement. It's time to stop fighting your staff, and start involving your staff!

BUT HOLD ON! As mentioned above, autonomy has to be earned through competence and trust. You don't simply turn over the keys to the castle to someone who you do not trust to exercise their own judgment and control. This is why I focused on setting expectations as the first principle. Employees need a lot of direction and instruction to competently perform their job. This might feel like more work on the front end, but the goal is for employees to succeed without having to constantly be managed. In other words, we want the extra work on the front end to result in less work on the back end. I call this "clearing the path" for employees to succeed. However; clearing the path requires more than just talking about expectations, leaders have to also commit to making sure employees are technically competent in their roles. That's the focus of the next chapter.

Chapter Four:
Coach Kevin

*"The growth and development of people
is the highest calling of leadership."*
– Harvey S. Firestone

You arrived to O'Donovan's 20 minutes late and find Robert and Tim already eating their meal.

"Hey, there's the good doctor!" Tim belts out when he sees you.

"Sorry I'm late gentlemen. A patient was asking some questions my staff couldn't answer and I got dragged into a lengthy discussion about multifocal contact lenses," you regretfully inform them. "Always happens right before lunch!"

"As long as you keep picking up the check, you can get here whenever you want!" Robert jokes. "How are things going in the practice?"

"I'm definitely seeing improvements in the staff's attitudes and performance. It's a work in progress, but everyone seems to have a much better understanding of their specific roles and responsibilities. My manager mentioned that lately she doesn't have to micromanage everyone. Micromanagement is probably something she learned from me. The challenge for me has been letting go of control. I've become very jaded in my thinking that anyone besides me can do the job right, which is why I've felt the need to control the entire process. I think they were very suspicious when I started asking for their input on ideas. Even more suspicious when I let them act on a few ideas. At first the staff was slow to respond, but that's slowly changing. Just yesterday one of my less vocal employees actually came to me with some ideas for social media marketing. It turns out that was one of her responsibilities at her last job. Who knew? For the most part, morale is up and the overall attitude in the practice has been more positive."

"Oh, this is fantastic!" Robert chimes in. You thought he was commenting on your newfound leadership skills, and then you notice he's staring at his corned beef on rye.

"So some good things are happening at the office," Robert directs his attention back to you.

"Yes, but I'm still a little frustrated with a few employees who keep making the same mistakes and doing unsatisfactory work."

"Can you give us some examples?" asks Robert.

"Most the issues involve taking too long to do tasks, a lot of billing mistakes and poor customer service."

"Tell me about your training process," Robert says.

"Well, we have a thirty day training process for new hires. For starters I'll admit it could use some improvement and I'm not even sure how much of it is handled. My manager is in charge of training, but she probably needs more training herself. She delegates some of it to other experienced employees but there's not much consistency in the process and I fear a lot of bad habits get passed down. I really should oversee it but I get busy seeing patients."

"What happens after the thirty days?" Robert asks.

"What do you mean?" you reply.

"Let me ask a question, what do your players call you?" asks Robert.

"Coach Kevin," you reply.

"What does your staff call you?" Robert inquires.

"They call me Doctor Bakon," you respond.

{long pause}

"Hold on, your name is Kevin Bacon?" Robert asks.

"Yes, my name is Kevin Bakon. Go ahead and have your laugh. For the record, it's Bakon with a K," you shoot back. You've lost count, but you're fairly certain you've explained this subtle spelling distinction over one million times.

"Whatever you say Doctor Kevin Bakon with a K," Robert quips. "Even though you've been sitting on that amusing nugget of information for the past two months, I'm going to let you off the hook. The person I want to talk about is Coach Kevin."

"Ok," you happily reply.

Robert looks at me and then glances over to Tim and asks when we made the decision to stop having baseball practice. Tim knows where this is going so he just smiles and keeps eating his fish & chips.

"I'm not following," you respond.

"Well, the kids you coach, they understand how to play baseball right? I mean, they know how to field and hit and pitch and they know that there are three outs in an inning, right? They understand the rules and the idea is to score more runs than the other team, right?" Robert asks.

"Well, um, yeah, but there's always something new they can learn. And just because they might understand the rules or how to play the game does not mean they should stop trying to improve their skills," you say. "Ok, I think I see where this is going."

"You see Mr. Bakon, in my world there's no end to training employees. Or to stay on theme, coaching people. There's always something new they can learn. There's always something old they could improve on. In fact, I've made a living coaching business owners. From my numerous years of experience I can tell you that there's really no point in business where you have "arrived". There is always something new to be learned and developed. So tell me Kevin, what happens after these thirty days of training that you offer new employees?"

"To be honest," you reply with a hint of embarrassment, "we don't really devote much time to developing our employees after the initial training period. It's not like we don't think it's important, we just all get busy with our own jobs and ongoing coaching was not a priority. I suppose a lack of time was the biggest obstacle."

"Ok," Robert replies with a tone of understanding. "That's probably the most common pushback I hear when I recommend an ongoing employee development program to my clients. We don't have time! Let me ask you this, when you weren't seeing patients last week what did you spend most of your time doing?"

"Let's see, accounts receivable has been a disaster. I've been working with my office manager to try and get that under control."

"Is that your office manager's responsibility?" Robert asks.

"No," you respond. "She used to do the billing but now we have another billing person who's been with us for two years but she makes a lot of mistakes."

"Has your manager ever provided any ongoing training or coaching with her?" Robert inquires. This prompts you to laugh. One of your office manager's favorite phrases is "she has worked here long enough to know how to do the job". Training new hires is her least favorite part of the job, and she is more likely to do another employee's job for them before offering additional training.

"What else did you do last week?" asks Robert.

"Looking back on last week, I had to deal with two angry patients who left negative online reviews. One was upset because we gave her the wrong information about her insurance benefits and another complained about the long wait time. It didn't help that neither employee showed any concern for the patient's complaint when they were in the office. I spent a lot of time on the phone trying to rectify the situation with the patients and even more time counseling the employees."

"Well," says Robert as he strokes his chin and stares off into the distance, "I agree, you don't have time for ongoing employee coaching and development. You're too busy fixing all the damage that has resulted from not coaching and developing your employees!"

Robert let that sink in for a moment and then continues. "You see, a commitment to employee development tends to be a bigger investment on the front end, but eventually you can begin to back away because they will have a much better grasp on how to submit a claim, how to handle patient complaints, how to navigate your EHR system and all other aspects of their job. You spent last week putting out fires that never should have happened. Don't you see Kevin, without a commitment to ongoing employee development you're spending MORE time managing your employees, not less."

As you listen to this, your mind goes to coaching your son's baseball team. You think to yourself how your biggest joy in coaching these kids is watching them get a little better with each practice and with each game. This only happens with ongoing coaching and development. Throughout the season you've watched this group of young men develop into very good ball players. Robert was right, there were a lot more demands earlier in the season as every kid required a great deal of attention, but as the season went on each individual kid did not require as much of your attention. The kids knew what to do and how to do it without requiring as much instruction and supervision. What would this baseball team look like if the coaches hadn't invested in their ongoing development? You knew the answer. It would look like your staff!

At this point you tap your finger on the table in thought. You've hesitated to mention finances up to this point, mostly out of embarrassment, but you decide to open up about this with Robert and Tim.

"There's something else," you reply still looking at your tapping fingers to avoid eye contact. "Money has become a real problem. Our sales are down and we're struggling to keep up with the bills. I did not envision that three years in we would be struggling financially. My wife has always been supportive but I'd be lying if I said this wasn't putting a strain on our marriage. I can't even keep up with my student loan payments. We are just paying the interest. I don't know what we're going to do."

After a long pause, Tim breaks the silence. "Listen Kevin, I know as well as anyone how hard it is to run a business. I went through a lot of the same things as you. It's impossible to completely separate the business from your personal life, they are intertwined and each directly impacts the other."

You listen and nod your head in agreement.

"Kevin, guess how long my training program used to be at the store," Tim taps on the table with a spoon and fork to create the sound of a drum roll. "30 days! Just like yours. From that point I expected my employees to basically know everything. All I had really prepared them for at that point was to stock shelves and process transactions. When competition moved into town and price became a bigger factor, our sales dropped drastically. We were doing nothing to differentiate ourselves from the competition. I couldn't do it all by myself. I knew it had to be a team effort."

That sounds familiar, you think to yourself.

"Lucas mentioned yesterday at practice that you're a runner," Tim continued.

"Yeah," you reply. "I ran a few half marathons in my younger days, but mostly 5Ks these days."

"Where did you get your last pair of running shoes?" Tim asks.

You put your hand over your mouth to muffle the sound as you mention a popular sporting goods franchise.

"I won't hold that against you," Tim responds while pointing a butter knife in your direction, "but I would like you to visit my store. Since we've made employee development a priority at Tim's Sporting Goods, I have to say I'm pretty proud of the results. No pressure to buy anything, but I want you to experience what we've created. Even in a competitive market, our sales and revenue are up. I know why, but I would rather show you than tell you."

You accept the invitation. Besides, you could use a new pair of running shoes.

Welcome to Tim's Sporting Goods

"Welcome to Tim's Sporting Goods!" a young man calls out as you enter. "My name is Josh. How can I help you?"

"Hi Josh, I'm here to look at some running shoes," you inform the smiling employee.

"Oh, sure," he responds. "Let me walk you back to the shoe department and introduce you to Sam."

As you round a corner, you find yourself surrounded by a very impressive selection of athletic shoes. A young lady walks up to you and politely introduces herself. Her name is Samantha, Sam for short. "How can I help you today, sir," she asks.

"I'm in the market for some new running shoes," you inform her.

"Oh, you're a runner. That's great! What kind of running do you do?" she asks.

"I do some 5 and 10Ks, but mostly just for leisure and exercise," you say. You choose not to tell her that it's also an outlet from all the stress of managing the practice.

After answering a few pertinent questions about your running habits that a shoe salesperson had never previously asked you, Sam asked you to take off your shoes and walk away from her. You thought this was a bit odd, but your bigger concern was whether your socks had any holes in them. No holes! Whew. As you walked away from Sam, she asked you to turn around and walk back to her. When you turned around she was on one knee staring at your feet.

"Wow!" she says. "You are really flat footed. I notice your current running shoes have a shallow arch. Do you have any problems with your back?"

"Do I have problems with my back?" you repeat. "You have no idea! Last month I had to cancel patients for two days when I couldn't get off the couch. It's been manageable for the most part but about once or twice a year it acts up. Some episodes are worse than others." Sam then had you do a few more activities like run in place and stand on your toes as she intently focused on your feet.

"I'm not surprised by the back problems," Sam remarks. "One of the main functions of feet is to provide stability to the entire upper body. Flat feet are usually a result of how the bones formed while growing. Because of the lack of an arch in each foot, the stability of the upper body is diminished. This puts extra strain on the back muscles. Essentially the back muscles have to work harder to support themselves. Do you do any stretches or physical therapy?" she asks.

"I've tried a few. I looked up a few exercises online but truthfully I wasn't sure what exercises I should be doing and which ones were safe."

"That makes sense," Sam responded. "Let's look at some shoes first. I would like you to start wearing a shoe with adequate arch support for your condition. We also have orthopedic inserts that I strongly recommend. These will give you even more arch support and also help absorb the shock from running on pavement. If you have a few minutes when we're done, I'm happy to show you some safe stretches you can do before running to stretch out the back muscles and hamstrings. The shoes will help but you also need to stretch before and after you run. The hamstrings are a major contributor to back pain. How does all that sound?"

"Sam," you reply, "that sounds great!"

As you sign your credit card receipt and start heading toward the exit, a voice in the distance shouts out "Sam's great isn't she? You should see her in action with track and field athletes!" You turn around to find Tim walking toward you.

"I've got to hand it to you partner, I just spent more on shoes and accessories than I've ever spent before, and it didn't even hurt. Well, maybe a little. Great place you have here! Sam did a great job!" you raved.

"Thanks, but it wasn't always like this. In fact, this is how I met Robert. He was a customer here, and not a very happy customer. Long before we had a commitment to employee development, Robert came in with his son to purchase some equipment for football – shoes, pads and helmet as I recall. I wasn't on the floor when he was here, but my employee came to my office after he walked out and said, "You wouldn't believe the jerk that was just here. He kept asking all these questions I didn't know and then asked me why he would buy anything from here when he could get it cheaper from a competitor." I dismissed the situation, but about a week later I received a letter from Robert. He described his experience and said that he wanted to support a local proprietor but we failed miserably at earning his business. Customer service was below average. The salesperson could not speak knowledgeably about the products we sold. We didn't have what he wanted in stock and could not tell him when we expected to receive it. I saw on the stationary he sent that he was a business consultant. I initially felt very insulted by this letter, but I tossed and turned that night thinking about what he said. The next morning I got up, made myself a cup of coffee, sat in my favorite chair and thought to myself... he's right! Later that day I called Robert. First I apologized for the service he received, and then I asked if we could talk."

You listen closely as you draw comparisons to Robert's experience and that of your typical patient. Is that how your patients feel about your team?

"With Robert's help, our culture is completely different now," Tim continues. "Sure, we still have a training process for new hires to train them on the basic skills they need to do the job, but it doesn't stop there. We are always in training mode! We have sales reps discuss their products at team meetings. We watch videos on improving customer service. I've sent my sales team to lectures on improving sales skills. Last week we had a chiropractor talk to the staff during lunch. We cross-train employees in different departments and encourage every team member to share new things they learn with other employees. I like to say we are always "pouring into" our employees. I can't expect Sam to deliver the caliber of service you experienced today without continuously developing her knowledge and abilities. The same goes for all my employees. What you see here is not a thirty day approach to staff training, it's a never-ending approach to staff training!"

"But how do you have time for all of that?" you asked.

"I don't have time NOT to do all of that!" Tim fired back. "Kevin, do you know what I was doing while you were out here with Sam? I was closing a deal with a local college to provide all of the football gear for their players. As owner and CEO of Tim's Sporting Goods, that's where I need to be spending my time – growing the business, not just managing it. If you walked in this store five years ago, you would have found me running around like a mad man putting out fires and trying to do everyone else's job. There was no time for anything else. My inventory folks were constantly making mistakes with ordering. My salespeople were not very good at selling. Our customer service was abysmal. Without a commitment to continually coaching and developing the team, my time was monopolized by all the problems that resulted from my neglect in adequately coaching them to do their job at a high level. I was spinning my wheels and going nowhere."

"But what if you spend all this time developing your employees and they leave?" you ask.

Tim laughed. "What if I don't spend time developing my employees and they stay? That's the question you should be asking. This all made sense to me when Robert learned that I coached my oldest son's football team and he asked me a question."

"What was the question?" you inquire.

"When did you stop having football practice?"

Lesson #3:
Develop your employees

Whenever I hear of employees who are underperforming or failing at their job, and I hear it often, my first thought goes to whether the employee is failing the practice or the practice is failing the employee. As discussed in chapter 2, setting clear job expectations is critical in getting employees to understand their responsibilities and perform at a high level, but this alone is not enough. Employees also need to be adequately trained in all aspects of their job. While most organizations have an initial training process for new hires, the companies known for delivering great service and developing high performing teams are continuously investing in their people.

The character Sam is based on a real person. I've struggled with back issues for much of my adult life, and years ago a friend suggested I visit a local shoe store. Within minutes it became clear why he offered this suggestion. The employees were all extremely skilled and knowledgeable about the products they sold. In the category of going "above and beyond", they were also very knowledgeable about the anatomy of the foot and how that impacted the rest of the body. With that knowledge, my salesperson was able to effectively communicate how and why the shoes she reco-mmended, along with an orthopedic insert for greater arch support, would be a good investment. True to the story, I spent more on shoes than I had ever previously spent. Why? Because I wasn't just paying for shoes anymore, I was paying for relief from back pain.

A bit of a revelation occurred when I was checking out. Intended as a compliment, I jokingly asked the salesperson if she was in podiatry school. I say jokingly because she clearly wasn't old enough to be in grad school. Her reply was, "No, they just train us really well." I asked her about their training process and learned about their employee development program, where continuous learning and advancement of skills was a priority. When you study most successful organizations known for great service and high performing teams, you will find a commitment to continuous employee development.

We're too busy!

Employee coaching, training and development seem to be something nobody wants to do. Is there a website that offers staff training? Are there classes I can send them to? Can *you* come to my practice and train the staff? I hear this often from consulting clients and read similar posts on chat boards and social media forums. Yes, there are outside resources for staff training, but when a solid internal system does not exist for employee development, the result tends to be a team that does not perform up to expectations. In some cases, there exists a team that performs well below expectations.

The pushback I often hear is that there is not enough time to commit to employee development. That's a fair point. Most optometry practices are small businesses with limited people and resources. But if you find that a lot of your time, or your manager's time, is monopolized by staff management issues (recurring mistakes, uncompleted tasks, patient complaints, etc.), ask yourself if this could have been avoided or at least minimized with more staff training. To use my shoe example, also consider if your sales are suffering from insufficient staff training. For me, that was the revelation I mentioned above. What would our sales look like if our opticians were as knowledgeable and skilled as this young shoe salesperson? Do your employees know how to effectively ask questions, learn about a patient's wants and needs and confidently discuss solutions that address the patient's unique problems? Or are they just looking up vision benefits and processing transactions?

If you haven't seen it, check out this short video summarizing Daniel Pink's bestselling book *Drive: The Surprising Truth About What Motivates Us*. Pink's research uncovered three factors that lead to better performance and greater personal satisfaction in the workplace. Interestingly, autonomy (covered in Chapter 3) was one factor. Another was mastery, or the urge to get better at something. Did you ever notice that people seem to bring a higher level of energy to the workplace when they are very skilled and knowledgeable about their job? Have you observed this among your own employees? It's no coincidence. Investing time into staff training and development often has a positive return on investment!

How long should training take?

How long should staff training take? 30 days? 90 days? Don't answer that! It's a trick question. The answer is that training should never end. Just like the baseball team Kevin coaches, there's always something new employees can learn. This could be a formal learning process like sending employees to an industry conference or asking a frame rep to do an in-office presentation. It could also be simple "teaching moments" like the one I had when I realized my techs were telling patients who asked what the air puff test is for to "ask the doctor". That doesn't exactly instill confidence in their knowledge, does it? That was my fault. I never taught the staff what the air puff test did. So I pulled them aside and spent a few minutes discussing how the non-contact tonometer worked, what the normal results were and how it helped us in the diagnosis and treatment of glaucoma. It was rewarding to hear the techs now proudly speak with confidence when patients asked about the test, as opposed to the very uninspiring "I'm not sure, just ask the doctor". I'm sure the patients were impressed as well. This might seem like a trivial example, but great customer service is often the culmination of a lot of little things that add up to a great overall experience. An experience like Kevin had at the sporting goods store!

Don't forget the soft skills!

An office manager once told me they were considering terminating a new employee because she didn't make eye contact with patients and had a habit of talking to patients with her back to them while she was multi-tasking. I asked if they had spoke with her about this. They had not. Training programs tend to focus on teaching the technical skills of a job, but often fail to address the soft skills like eye contact, body language and how to effectively communicate. From a customer service standpoint, it's usually the soft skills that people remember. Consumers of any business assume employees will know 'how' to do their job, what they remember is the manner is which they did their job. Don't expect employees to naturally deliver in the soft skills area. Teach it! If you want your staff to deliver exceptional customer service, like Sam, you have to train the soft skills as well. Make that part of your ongoing employee development program. Remember, the goal is not perfection; it's continuous improvement. In a service industry, your people are your #1 asset. Water them like plants!

Next steps:

Is your approach to training and coaching haphazard and inconsistent? Do you delegate this to less than competent employees who potentially need more training themselves? Do you continue to develop and invest in your employees beyond the initial training or "onboarding" process?

Based on your answers to the above questions, I encourage you to introduce more structure and consistency into your employee training and development process. A haphazard approach allows for too many misunderstandings, poor practices and bad habits to get pushed down to new hires. Start by developing an employee training manual. A good time to create this is when you're training new hires. Simply document the steps required to perform required tasks and turn this into a manual. Do this for each position. This serves as a consistent method for training new hires (the way YOU want them trained) and also a manual that employees can refer back to. This can remain a working document that can be changed and updated as positions and responsibilities change. Be patient with new hires and be willing to revisit training for employees who are struggling with certain aspects of their job. If you're feeling techy, you can create short "how-to" videos for new hires. Visuals can be more impactful and memorable than text or verbal explanations. Provide trainees with a notebook to keep notes during the training process and get comfortable asking trainees to repeat back to you or demonstrate what they've been taught to ensure that they clearly understand. As discussed, the goal is to "clear the path" for new hires to succeed without having to constantly be managed. From a leadership standpoint, the best managers and supervisors ultimately make their own jobs easier, not harder!

Chapter Five:
The Self-Improvement Fallacy

"Everybody is a genius. But if you judge a fish by its ability to climb a tree, it will live its whole life feeling stupid."
— Matthew Kelly

Tim and Robert almost didn't recognize you as you walked into O'Donovan's for the latest round of advice, answers and amusing anecdotes. Dressed head to toe in full running gear, including the new shoes you purchased from Tim's Sporting Goods, you headed toward the usual booth.

"Was this your idea?" Robert asks while pointing at you and looking at Tim. "I don't remember ever suggesting casual Tuesdays at the office."

"I feel alive gentlemen!" you pronounce with vigor and optimism that Robert and Tim have not seen up to this point.

"What's gotten into you?" Tim asks. "Nice shoes by the way!"

"Thanks!" you reply. "I know this great place on the north side of town called Tim's."

"I'll have to check it out sometime," Tim replies. "So to what reason do we owe this upbeat version of Dr. Bakon?"

"Well, I have to admit things are going better in the practice. Better teamwork, less mistakes and improved morale. Employees are taking more initiative and ownership in their roles. I don't feel as stressed as I previously did, feeling that I was the only one who could solve all the problems I was facing. It's not perfect by any stretch, but it's better. It's noticeably better!"

"Perfect?" Tim questions. "Perfect is never the goal. As Robert will tell you, perfect can become the enemy of very good. I've found steady and continuous improvement to be a much more realistic goal for my stores. When you study most successful organizations, you will find a leadership team that continuously drives improvements in the company, along with a strong aversion to simply maintaining the status quo. Sometimes these attempts at improvements result in failure, but the top organizations learn from these mistakes. I would say this approach is very much aligned with what has made my stores successful. I sometimes joke with other business owners that the reason Tim's Sporting Goods has grown while competitors have gone out of business is because we've made more mistakes than they have. Not everybody gets that, but successful business owners can usually relate. The point is that we've embraced change, and even though we've made our share of mistakes, we are committed to always trying new things and not getting stuck in trying to maintain the status quo. When everyone else is crying about big box competitors and online sporting good retailers, we are looking for ways to adapt and improve. If you own *any* business these days and you're not doing this, you're likely in for a real struggle!"

You nod your head in agreement as you consider the similarities between Tim's remarks about the sporting goods industry and the eye care industry.

"Now Robert here would probably tell you I made too many mistakes early on, but I find that I make far fewer mistakes now as I've learned to involve my team. As we've discussed, business owners have to make a lot of high-level decisions and will likely make better decisions when they have more information. That requires a willingness, along with some humility, to acknowledge that you don't have all the answers. You'll likely go much farther as part of a team than you will as an individual."

"Uh um," Robert loudly clears his throat.

"Oh yeah," Tim responds. "All that and the help of a great business consultant!"

"Well thank you good sir!" Robert graciously replies.

"But enough about me," Tim switches gears. "What's with the outfit?"

"Oh," you reply. "Speaking of improvement, because the staff has been doing a much better job I decided to reward them with a paid afternoon off. And since I'm not seeing patients this afternoon, I decided to go for a run. And by the way, I want to mention again how impressed I was with the service I got at your store. Especially Sam! She was great!"

"Thanks! I appreciate the kind words," Tim replies. "Fortunately Sam is still with us. About six months ago she handed in her resignation."

"Really?" you reply in a tone of surprise. "She seems to love her job. She's very good at sales."

"She is," Tim agrees, "except she wasn't in sales at the time. She was a cashier."

"A cashier?" you reply. "Well, I'm sure she was good at that too, but it seems like a mistake to have someone so charismatic and personable not utilized on the sales floor. To be honest, with finances being somewhat tight lately I really didn't intend to spend as much as I did, but by taking the time to understand my personal needs and effectively communicate the reasons to invest in higher quality products, I was sold!"

"Great observations, and I agree Kevin." Tim responds. "But believe it or not, she wasn't that great of a cashier. As part of her exit interview, I asked about her reasons for leaving. She was fairly blunt in telling me she was bored in her position. Being a cashier at Tim's Sporting Goods is very transactional. There is not much opportunity to connect with people. There were also some weekly financial reports that had to be completed which she dreaded. Her mathematical skills and attention to detail weren't strengths of hers and she tended to make a lot of mistakes on these reports, causing excess time to be wasted as my managers had to frequently double check her work. She told me her previous job was a salesperson at a jewelry store where she was frequently 'employee of the month'. She discussed how she loved helping the customers pick out the perfect piece of jewelry. She had unfortunately lost her mother on the day of her parent's wedding anniversary and took a special interest in helping men pick out anniversary gifts for their spouse. At some point in this exit interview, the conversation took an odd but enlightening turn. We started talking about jewelry. I told Sam I had a wedding anniversary coming up and she lit up! Over the next 20 minutes I learned more about diamonds than I've ever known. As she was mid sentence telling me about the 4 Cs (that's diamond talk for cut, clarity, color and carat), I held up my hand and told her I had an idea. I asked her, and by ask I mean beg, to withdrawal her resignation and move to the sales floor. It took a little convincing and a small raise but she agreed to give it a try. From the first day in her new role she has been a star. She's a completely different employee! She brings a lot of enthusiasm and energy to the role that has been infectious with the rest of the team, not to mention great for sales! At her last performance review she mentioned how much happier she is coming to work."

"That's interesting," you observe. "As I've strived to improve my leadership skills, I find that some people are more receptive than others. Maybe I would be more effective if employee's strengths were aligned with their roles and responsibilities. I tend to want to fix people's weaknesses."

"That's exactly what many employers try to do, fix weaknesses." Robert chimes in. "Don't get me wrong, we all have our strengths and we all have our weaknesses, and certainly some weaknesses would benefit from some additional training and coaching, but in general people are much more engaged in their roles and bring a higher level of energy to the workplace when their job duties are aligned with their strengths and interests. When you are dealing with an underperforming employee it is certainly possible that you made a poor hire, but it's also possible that you simply have this employee in the wrong role. In Tim's case, he had a standout salesperson hidden behind a cash register. Once he took the time to understand what Sam's strengths were, he made a realignment."

"These days I spend less time trying to fix weaknesses." Tim interjects. "I, along with my managers, make a point to observe our employees. We note people's areas of strengths. This could be a gregarious personality, commitment to teamwork, attention to detail, leadership attributes, or any other quality that would translate to a valuable asset for the company. We also discuss this in our one-on-ones with employees. We ask what they like and dislike about their jobs. We've worked to establish a high trust environment so employees will feel comfortable voicing their honest feedback. Through these discussions we learn about each employee and how we can make Tim's Sporting Goods a great place to work. This might sound like it's strictly for the benefit of the employees, but it's not! For Tim's, it's led to better production, higher morale and lower turnover."

Later that day you will see this approach played out on the baseball diamond as you observe the team playing their final game of the year. There is a reason that every player plays the position he does – the player's strengths are best suited for that role. Albeit a less athletic comparison, why would the workplace be any different? As you watch your fastest player chase down and catch a ball in center field that looked certain to be a multiple base hit, you make the decision to do a more effective job observing and understanding your employees strengths, and hopefully spend less time trying to fix everyone's weaknesses – a job you've found increasingly frustrating with less than optimal returns.

Lesson #4:
Now, discover your (*employee's*) strengths

In the bestselling book *Now, Discover Your Strengths* by Marcus Buckingham and Donald O. Clifton, strengths are defined as a combination of talent, knowledge and skills.

Talent is naturally occurring patterns of thought, feeling or behavior that can be productively applied. Usually talents come so natural to us that we don't recognize them as talents. In fact, sometimes talents come so easily that we make the mistake of assuming everyone can do the same things.

Knowledge is facts and lessons learned. Knowledge can be factual (knowing product features or protocols, etc.) or experiential (learned through experience). As we learned in the employee development chapter, a successful employee-training program must go beyond the initial new hire training process.

Skills are the steps of an activity. Skills are necessary to perform a task but will not necessarily allow you to excel at it. For example, you may learn the basic steps of selling a pair of glasses, but without the natural sales talent, you will never be great at it.

Knowledge and skills can be developed and refined, but without talent it's unlikely that an employee will be able to consistently perform at a high level. For example, if the role requires an employee to exhibit leadership or empathy or assertiveness and he or she lacks the natural talent for one of these, the employee will likely struggle in this role. As an employer or manager, much of your attention will be diverted to fixing weaknesses (damage control) as opposed to employee development.

Recently I consulted a client who promoted her lead optician to office manager. By all accounts, this employee was a stellar optician. ABO certified, extremely knowledgeable and skilled. The decision was made to promote this individual to office manager. To the OD's surprise, the former optician struggled mightily in this new role. She was impatient with other less experienced employees, often doing their work for them out of frustration as opposed to developing their knowledge and skills. She had difficulty relating to others who lacked her optical talents, and her abrasive and at times condescending attitude caused others to avoid approaching her with questions or clarifications. This led to problems when she was not at work as other employees made frequent mistakes since they were not adequately trained. The new office manager would often say, "They've worked here long enough – they should know how to do their job!" Essentially, she didn't want to be bothered with these distractions. It became clear that this individual lacked the leadership talents necessary to be successful in this role. My consulting client was asking, "How do I *fix* this person?" I had to inform her that she likely promoted someone who would never excel in this role, at least not consistently. She possessed the skills and knowledge necessary to do the job, but she lacked the leadership talent critical to this role. It is possible to promote someone right into incompetence.

Let's look at this from the opposite side. What qualities make someone a good office manager? For starters, I'll acknowledge that there is more than one effective leadership style, but having worked with numerous office managers I've come to recognize a few commonalities among those that succeed in this challenging role. I'll mention two examples. They always put the needs of the practice above their title (more results-driven than ego-driven), and they provide consistent feedback and coaching to their team to develop their skills and abilities. These are the managers who call me on the phone or pull me to the side at conferences to discuss ways to improve the practice. In other words, they want to *lead* their team to success. In the case of the manager discussed above, she was more concerned about herself than the success of the practice. This wasn't as apparent when she was an optician, but became apparent as her new role required leadership talents. The leadership talents inherent in the successful managers I mentioned did not come natural to this struggling manager, and it's unlikely they ever will. It's possible for her to continue to develop her managerial skills and knowledge, but without managerial talent she will likely continue to deliver a subpar performance.

While many employers spend a disproportionate amount of time trying to fix their employee's weaknesses, your employee's greatest potential for growth is in their areas of strength. As an organization, try to match each employee's strengths to his or her position and roles at work. Consider this when you are hiring for a position, but also consider realignment with your current staff if you feel certain employee's positions or responsibilities are not aligned with their strengths. From a motivational standpoint, employees will bring a higher level of energy to the workplace when they are utilizing their talents. Studies show that people who are able to pursue their passions at work experience *flow*, a euphoric state of mind that is five times more productive than the norm. In sports, they call this being in the *zone*!

But it's their job!

Can I challenge a comment I hear frequently? "That's his/her job!" A client once called me about an employee who had completed her first 90 days of employment and they were considering terminating her. The reason was because she frequently made mistakes on a routine administrative task. The doctor told me that everyone needed to know how to do this task. Apparently she had been coached and counseled on this but continued to make mistakes. The doctor quietly wondered if she had a learning disability. When I asked about her other attributes, all I heard was positivity. She was very friendly and charismatic, a great team player, the patients liked her and she generally wanted to improve in her role. I told the doctor that I was struggling to agree with him that terminating this employee was the right thing to do. "But this is part of her job!" After we talked this through, he opened up to the idea that maybe he could salvage this employee by shifting her responsibilities to areas that leveraged her strengths and avoided her weaknesses. We decided she would be a better fit working with patients on the retail side. Her talent was her charismatic and outgoing personality. Reluctantly at first, he decided to stop requiring her to do this administrative task and delegated it to other employees. Over time, this led him to rethink each employee's roles and responsibilities. The bottom line... let's double down on people's strengths and stop asking them to do things they're never going to be good at! I understand that in most small to mid-size businesses there is typically some cross-training and employees need to wear multiple hats, but instead of getting locked into rigid job descriptions where failure is defined by not being great at everything, let's look for ways to be flexible when assigning primary roles and responsibilities to employees. In baseball terms, there's a reason the fastest player plays center field and the pitcher bats last.

Next steps:

If you're not already doing this, start observing your employees. Great leaders are great observers of people. They are always looking for strengths in the people they lead and striving to put them in positions that exploit these strengths. The common practice of assigning responsibilities that exploit weaknesses only sets up the employee for failure and results in a lot more work for the manager or employer. If you've ever coached a sport, this comes natural. The slow kid on the team who can crush a baseball would not be a great center fielder, but would likely be very effective hitting in the cleanup position. If you don't know what that means, then start watching more baseball. It's a great sport!

In addition to observing your employees and identifying their strengths and weaknesses, I suggest you also try this. In your one-on-ones ask them what they enjoy about their position and what they dislike about it. Strengths and interests tend to go hand in hand. We usually take greater joy in doing things we are good at and bring a higher level of energy to these tasks. In the case of Sam, she liked helping people, not completing financial reports! If possible, consider shifting responsibilities to allow people to spend more time doing work they enjoy. There's absolutely no upside to a dull, boring workplace. Who says a job can't be enjoyable?

Lastly I'll mention there are commercially available personality tests you could administer to current employees and also candidates you are considering hiring. The information from these tests can tell you a lot about someone's strengths and weaknesses and take much of the guesswork out of the process. I once took a personality test and was very impressed with the results. The summarized results, based on my answers to questions, looked like my mom and wife had got together and wrote a few paragraphs about me – the good and the bad! I remember laughing when I read it and thinking, "yep, that's me!"

Chapter Six:
The Setback

"Give someone responsibility and they will do their best. Make them accountable and they will do even better."
— Simon Sinek

Today will be your last lunch date with Robert and Tim. You wish that wasn't the case, as some problems have crept back into the organization. For some reason, Robert insisted after the last meeting that you wait six months before joining them again and hearing of the final lesson. You pause before opening the door to O'Donovan's Pub, knowing you will have to report that some of the progress made the first few months has not stuck.

"Did you miss me?" you ask as you take your seat at the regular booth.

"I'm sorry, who are you?" Robert replies.

"Very funny," you reply. "Where's Tim?"

"Tim called and said he'd be late. He got held up at the store."

As you stare off into the distance, a rare moment of awkward silence fills the air. You know Robert is about to ask you about the practice and you're not quite sure what to say. You fear disappointing your mentor. Maybe Tim will show up soon and that discussion can be delayed with some small talk.

"So how have things been going with the practice since I last saw you?" Robert asks. No small talk.

"Well, let me start by saying this journey has been very enlightening and I've learned a ton about managing and leading people. There have certainly been drastic improvements in my staff's performance, leading to drastic improvements in my business. I now see ownership and leadership with a fresh perspective."

"But?" Robert asks after a long pause.

Trying to find the right words, you blurt out "It didn't stick!"

"What do you mean it didn't stick?" Robert asks.

"Well, everything seemed to be improving in the beginning. Sure, there were some days better than others, but overall I really sensed a turning point in the office where employees were more energized and committed to their jobs. There was greater clarity on their roles and responsibilities. They seemed to react positively to being given more involvement in decisions and independence in how they performed their job. My manager and I have been more proactive in developing the employees, and we've been more observant with individual strengths and weaknesses and tried to take this into consideration when assigning roles and responsibilities."

"And you've seen some of this hard work go to waste?" asks Robert.

"Yes!" you proclaim. "It's frustrating! Things are certainly better than the first time we sat down for lunch, but I expected the momentum to continue in a positive direction. The past few months it feels like we've been going in the wrong direction. Old habits are returning. Performance is dipping. And worst of all our revenues, which were trending up at an impressive rate when we began this process, are trending back down. Maybe I'm just not meant to own a business. I thought at this point I would be as optimistic about the future as Tim, but I feel like I'm slowly being pulled back into the stress and chaos I felt before."

Expecting a sympathetic response from Robert, he stares emotionless at you for a moment before asking a very stern and direct question. "Tell me about consequences."

"What do you mean cons…?"

"Consequences!" Robert fires back before you get the word out of your mouth. "What consequences were there for the employees who did not meet performance expectations that were clearly communicated to them?"

You had not seen this side of Robert before and found yourself really hoping Tim would show up soon to break the tension. "Umm" was the only phrase you could muster up.

"Tell me about meetings you've had with employees to discuss performance." Robert commands.

"We still have our weekly team meetings," you reply.

"Not *team* meetings," responds Robert. "I'm talking about private, one-on-one meetings where you ask employees to report on their performance."

{long, uncomfortable pause}

As your intimidation slowly turns to aggravation over this confrontational line of questioning, you ask, "What is this, an interrogation?"

"No Kevin," Robert responds with a slight hint of a smile. "It's lesson five."

Still a bit confused, but happy to feel the tension lift, Tim rapidly approaches the table. "Did I miss the part where you get all serious?"

"All done," Robert remarks.

"Damn!" Tim responds. "That was my favorite part of lesson five."

"Kevin, do you know why I asked you to wait six months before meeting up with us again?" asks Robert.

"I can't say I'm one hundred percent certain," you reply.

Culture change in any organization happens slowly. It develops slowly and it changes slowly. I wanted you to see what could happen over an extended time if you failed to hold employees accountable for results."

There it was. Lesson five… holding people accountable.

"You see," Robert continues, "you can do everything we discussed in the first four lessons – you can set clear expectations, allow for autonomy, coach and develop your staff and put them in positions of strength - but if you don't hold your employees accountable for desired outcomes, it's very likely that people will resort back to their old ways. The old culture, the one you worked so hard to improve, will begin to resurface."

"Ok," you say in agreement. "Obviously that's happened. But how do I hold people accountable? Follow them around all day looking over their shoulder to make sure they're doing their work and doing it right? I thought I was supposed to allow some autonomy in the workplace and not micro-manage people?"

"What you just described sounds like a terrible place to work! I wouldn't want to work for a boss who was always looking over my shoulder and pointing out everything I did wrong," says Robert.

"So what's the secret?" you ask. "What's the magic formula for motivating people and getting people to continue to perform at a high level?"

"There's no magic formula Kevin. In fact, you're probably already doing it in other areas of your life. Let me ask about your kids. They're in school, right? I'm certain you've set certain expectations around scholastic performance. I'm sure you've been involved in teaching them by helping with schoolwork. You've probably given them some freedom to complete school projects using their own ideas, and you've likely encouraged them to take classes and pursue extra-curricular activities that align with their strengths and interests."

You nod your head in agreement.

"Do your hold your kids accountable for their school performance?" Robert asks.

"Of course!" you reply.

"Got it!" Robert says. "So you follow them around at school looking over their shoulder during class and remarking whenever they make a mistake or perform below expectations?"

"Well, no." you respond. "Every month the teachers send home a progress report and my wife and I sit the kids down to go over their performance."

"What happens if they bring home bad marks?" Robert asks.

"I have to say their grades have been very good. I suspect much of it has to do with knowing in advance that they will have to look mom and dad in the eye and report back to us on their performance."

And there it was. Accountability! It made perfect sense when you heard yourself say it. Accountability is getting people to perform in a way in which they know in advance they will have to "account" for their performance at a later date. That's why Robert grilled you with questions about the last time you met with employees to review their performance. This had not taken place. And the truth is you had not always met with your kids to review their school performance. A few years ago you and Katie were so overwhelmed with the practice that you began neglecting your kids school activities. Their grades slowly began to drop, and it wasn't until you began meeting with them individually and requiring them to answer for their grades and progress reports that you started to see improvement. Once they knew in advance they were going to have to answer for their school performance, they took their schoolwork much more serious. Had you not done that, it's likely their grades would have continued to slide – similar to your employee's performance over the past few months."

You didn't realize you were mumbling these words to yourself and as your mind drifts from your parenting skills back to the present, you look up to see Robert and Tim beaming with wide smiles.

"What?" you ask.

"Our baby's all grown up!" Tim responds pretending to wipe a tear from his eye.

Robert then raises his iced tea to celebrate the moment. "Kevin," Robert states, "here's to a bright future." As the sound of three glasses clink together, you think back to an earlier comment you made to Tim wishing your employees were as coachable as the kids on the team you coached. You now realize the obstacle to success was not the people you were hiring, it was you! Every lesson you learned from Robert and Tim required YOU to take action, even if that action was parting ways with an employee who proved to be uncoachable and recalcitrant after diligently applying these five principles. You feel a renewed sense of optimism knowing that you have more control over your success than you previously thought, but you also feel a sense of anxiety knowing that you are the one responsible for this success.

As you finish saying your goodbyes to Robert and Tim, Robert leaves you with one final piece of advice. "Kevin," Robert says. "I've worked with business owners who blame everything under the sun for their failures. They blame the economy, new technology, competition, and a host of other external factors. The one person they don't blame is themself. All these lessons have been geared toward becoming a better leader, and leaders in any organization do not only hold others accountable, more importantly they hold themselves accountable. Don't forget that."

"I certainly won't," you reply.

Lesson #5:
Accountability

Are you terrible at holding people accountable? "Terrible" is not my word, it was the word chosen in a 2012 Harvard Business Review article titled "One Out of Every Two Managers is Terrible at Accountability". In a study of 5,400 high level managers, nearly 50% rated themselves poorly on the item, "Hold people accountable – firm when they don't deliver." Out of all the leadership responsibilities of managers, the most commonly dodged responsibility is holding people accountable.

Without establishing a mechanism of accountability in the workplace, it's much more likely that your attempts at building an empowered, engaged work force will fail. You can be clear with expectations, allow for autonomy, develop employees and put them in positions of strength, but there still remains a human condition known as 'resistance to change'. If you're never asking employees to change, there's less need for accountability. Just show up and do your job. That's called maintaining the status quo. But if you seek a culture of continuous improvement, that will require change. And it will also require holding people accountable for their roles in contributing to these improvements.

Without accountability, it's very easy for people to slip back into old ways and habits without fear of consequences. These are the practices that will say, "We tried it for a while but the staff went back to doing it the old way." When I ask about the consequences – crickets!

How do I hold people accountable?

Discussions around employee accountability almost always provoke this question. How do I hold people accountable? Unfortunately, there tends to be a perception around this topic that conjures up images of a dictatorial, draconian work environment. I hope by now you see the limitations put on a workforce that operates in a micromanaged environment. You may get people's compliance, but you won't get their energy or commitment. Obviously a micromanaged, highly supervised work environment would be the opposite extreme of an autonomous, independent work environment. Accountability does not require organizational leaders to follow people around constantly supervising their work and pointing out every time they make a mistake or fall short of expectations. There may be some industries or work environments where that is necessary, but in a service industry like optometry this will likely stifle the work performance of the employees and lead to high turnover and low morale.

When you think of accountability, think of "answerability". Accountability is established when people perform their job knowing in advance they will have to answer for their performance at a later date. To pull a term from the corporate world, this involves asking employees to "report" to a superior. In most optometry practices this will either be the practice owner or a manager. Remember, this comes after leadership has clearly communicated expectations and the employee has been given the tools, training and resources to succeed. Accountability is reinforced when the employee has to report on outcomes and progress. When appropriate, this can be part of a staff meeting agenda, but there's also value to meeting with individual employees in a private setting.

One-on-one meetings

I think regular staff meetings are very valuable and should be a regular part of your weekly routine, but staff meetings have their shortcomings. It's easy for the underperformers to hide out at staff meetings. They can sit in the back and remain quiet while the leaders and high performers dominate the conversation. Less vocal team members may be too intimidated to speak up publicly. Also, staff meetings are not the appropriate forum for discussing individual performance problems. Most of the time owners or managers are scheduling one-on-one discussions with an employee, it is to reprimand him or her for some aspect of their job performance that they are dissatisfied with. In many cases, this uncomfortable meeting could have been avoided – along with all the fires and drama that preceded it – simply by management being more engaged in the performance expectations of the employee. This cannot happen in the shadows. It requires frequent and high-quality one-on-one communication with all of your employees.

In 2009, statisticians at Google embarked on a plan to determine the top habits of highly effective managers. Through extensive data mining involving performance reviews, feedback surveys and nominations for top-manager awards, they determined that the most effective managers were those who periodically made time to meet with employees one-on-one. These meetings allowed for clarifying expectations, answering questions, listening to the employee's ideas and puzzling through problems by asking questions, not dictating answers. All these issues are very important and consistent with the principles put forth in this book, but another purpose of these meetings is to provide candid feedback on performance issues.

I recommend not making assumptions or jumping to conclusions with low-performers. Review goals and expectations and ask the employee to report on the status of their work. If he or she is failing to meet expectations, ask why. Sometimes there are valid reasons. Perhaps the employee needs more training, was unclear on priorities, or is so overwhelmed with other tasks that they lack the time to get all their work done. This is where leadership steps in to provide additional support for the employee, not a reprimand.

But let's look at a different scenario. You've been clear with expectations and provided all the tools, training and resources for the employee to succeed, but they are still performing below expectations. This is where accountability is necessary. Where accountability is lacking, you cannot expect the situation to improve. Requiring employees to report on their performance on a regular basis is likely to get results. In general, people get uncomfortable having to look their boss in the eye and continually explain why they are failing to perform at the level expected of them. In the story we used the analogy of kids not wanting to explain poor grades to their parents. Ideally we want both kids *and* employees to volunteer their best efforts, but the reality is some people need a process to keep them performing at an acceptable level. This can't be stressed enough – where accountability lacks, underperformers will thrive – at underperforming!

What if the performance doesn't improve?

That's a possibility. Accountability only establishes conse-quences, but doesn't guarantee results. Some studies have found that the number one reason new hires fail at the job they were hired to do is lack of coachability. These are the employees who have been given the tools, training and resources to succeed and for whatever reason choose not to. At this point you have a decision to make, is this something we can live with or would we be better off parting ways with this individual? If you're diligent in your efforts at holding employees accountable, it's likely they will either start showing improvement (if for no other reason than to avoid this uncomfortable conversation with their boss), or they will make the decision to leave on their own. Not all turnover is bad.

Next steps:

Hopefully it's become clear throughout this book why I think frequent and ongoing communication with employees is so critically important, both as a team and one-on-one. You may or may not have regular staff meetings, but if you're like many practices you're probably not carving out time to meet individually with each employee on a regular basis to review their job performance. And if high-level feedback is only offered every 12 months at annual reviews, the employee problems that develop often stem from the issue at hand — a lack of communication!

Set up regular one-on-one meetings with each employee. At a minimum, I suggest quarterly. This can certainly be delegated to a trusted and competent office manager. Reassure employees that the goal of these meetings is to help them succeed in their roles. It's an opportunity for leaders to listen as well. As important as communication is, good communicators are even better listeners. They first seek to learn about people and situations before providing feedback and direction. What challenges are they facing? What obstacles are in their way? How can I support my team in achieving our goals? One-on-one meetings provide a safe environment for employees to discuss matters that they might avoid discussing in a public setting. In the words of Stephen R. Covey, "Seek first to understand, then to be understood". Wise advice for leaders!

On the topic of accountability, employees need to also be clear that they will be expected to answer for performance and outcomes at these meetings. As kids, why did we work hard in school to get good grades? Because we had to look mom and dad in the eye each grading period and answer for our scholastic performance. There was accountability! It's very similar with employees. It's a leaders responsibility to set clear goals and expectations, provide adequate training and development, put people in positions that leverage their talents and be willing to involve them in the process, but once that is done employees need to be held accountable for results.

If accountability is lacking or in some cases non-existent, the chance of successfully motivating employees and creating an engaged, high-performing team (the focus of this book) is greatly diminished. Accountability is the glue that holds it all together. As mentioned in the intro, this book provides the information. Consistently executing these principles is up to you.

You're up to bat!

Conclusion

How do I motivate people?

That's where we began, with a quest to uncover the best ways to motivate people. Here is a conclusion I've come to – it's hard to motivate people! It's hard to motivate ourselves, let along others. If it were easy we would all be millionaires with 6-pack abs. Motivation implies that people care, and it's hard to make people care! Think about this in you own life. Most of the things that motivate you are likely things you personally care about, right? Whether it's growing a business, running a marathon or coaching your kid's baseball team, the things that truly motivate you are things that you genuinely care about. Sure, some employees are naturally driven and self-motivated, but expecting this same level of commitment from all employees will likely leave you frustrated and disappointed. This is where leadership matters! And as a leader, you will likely have more long-term success altering the work environment than you will have trying to alter the employee. That was the focus of this book.

Spend less time trying to change people, and more time changing your work environment. Many of the people we hire do not need a pep talk; they need a process!

It's hard to find good people!

Yes, that's probably true. But the next time you're considering parting ways with that underperforming employee, ask yourself if the employee failed the practice, or the practice failed the employee. People are flawed and this book won't help you eliminate employee failure, but I hope that proactively implementing these principles allows you to improve overall staff performance and as a result experience higher revenues, less stress and more personal time. It's my observation that you'll get there much faster with the help of a great team than you will by yourself.

My a-ha moment

Someone once asked me about the #1 thing I've learned consulting with optometry practices. My answer was "I've learned to be a better listener". Early on in my new role I tended to offer information before taking the time to fully understand the situation and the people involved. On the initial call with a new consulting client, the practice owner will often mention things like declining revenues, inventory management or staff challenges as reasons for hiring a consultant. But as the conversations continue and a level of trust develops, you often learn the *real* reasons that practice owners want help with their business. I'll hear stories of wanting to spend more time with their kids, have less stress, or take their wife on a vacation. Your business is an extension of your personal life and as we saw with Dr. Kevin, the two are not mutually exclusive. The characters in this book were fictitious, but for many practice owners the storyline is very real.

3 years later

It's been three years since your lunch meetings with Robert and Tim. Things have changed dramatically since these meetings. You still experience challenges with managing staff. It's not perfect. It's not easy. But it's better. In fact, it's much better. By implementing Robert's suggestions into your approach of managing staff, the result has been better teamwork, less turnover, higher production and happier employees. You hadn't realized how much time you were spending on managing the inadequacies of a poor staff. The truth is, it was a lack of leadership that led to all the extra time and effort involved with managing. With a renewed commitment to effective leadership and staff management, you found that you and your manager actually spend less time having to manage people, not more. There was more work on the front end, but the payoff was less work (and problems) on the back end.

The final pitch

On this night you've invited your wife Katie out to dinner at a familiar spot – O'Donovan's Pub. You called ahead to reserve the same booth you both sat in when you originally hashed out plans to open a private practice. After you each ordered your meals, you slide an envelope over to her side of the table. She looks at the envelope with curiosity, and then looks at you with a suspicious grin. After a moment of contemplation, she picks up the envelope and opens it. It contains a letter from your student loan lender informing you that the balance has been paid off on your one remaining loan. In that same envelope she discovers two round trip tickets to the Bahamas.

As you raise your wine glass to offer a cheer, you realize she is crying. In some ways this ends a long journey, and in others it begins a new journey.

Cheers!

EYE

ON

LEADERSHIP

5-Week Leadership Training Course

Week 1: Let's Be Clear

Welcome to Week 1 of Eye on Leadership, a 5-week course designed to make you a better leader!

In this course, you can expect to get:

- A vision of what it means to be a great leader
- A powerful framework for solving staff management problems
- Practical leadership skills you can begin using tomorrow
- A specific process and action-plan to get you started

In short, you will get the mind-set, skill-set and tool-set necessary to create a motivated and engaged team and achieve your goals.

Lesson 1: Let's Be Clear!

Leadership begins with clarity. And as practice owner or manager, you are a leader! The best leaders are often credited with being great communicators; in terms of communicating expectations to employees to create a unified team that understands the goals of the organization and what they need to do to achieve these goals. If team members are not clear on their specific responsibilities and expected outcomes, how can they be expected to succeed in their roles?

The attached book, *Eye on Leadership*, will serve as the handbook for this course. This is the story of a practice owner who turned his practice around in 3 years using many on the leadership principles that will be presented to you over the next 5 weeks. **For this week, read the Introduction and Chapters 1 and 2.** When you finish that, complete the assignments below.

Week 1 Assignments:

1. Clarify the Vision

I want you to envision what you want your practice to look like in 3 - 5 years. How many staff members will you have? How much revenue will you generate? How big will your office be? How many days will you see patients? Consider your personal life as well. How much time off will you have? What will you do with that time off? Now write this vision down on paper. This is YOUR dream so don't hold back! Be very specific! If you're in a leadership role but not the owner, then revise this per your role and responsibilities. Managers often play a significant role in the growth of a practice. Write down your vision from a manager's perspective. It's ok if this changes and evolves over time, but it's important that you have a meaningful vision worth pursuing. Clarity involves having a clear vision of WHAT you want and HOW you're going to get it.

Why 3 - 5 years? Generally speaking, if your vision and goals are too far out or feel too unrealistic, you will be less likely to pursue them. On the same hand, success does require patience. It's the discipline that comes with doing the small things consistently that often leads to massive success down the road. Three to five years is a nice sweet spot for me, but you can adjust that if you like. The important thing is to have a vision that excites you!

On a side note, I often ask new consulting members about their vision and goals for their practice. Consistently, the more successful practices are quick to describe a vision with greater clarity and detail. I find the less successful practices need a few moments to ponder this, and then reply with a somewhat vague description. I suspect their focus has been on current circumstances and not future goals. High performing leaders have a great ability to focus on the future and what they want to create. When you and the people you lead become disconnected from the future, enthusiasm wanes and performance declines. No goals, no growth. No clarity, no change.

2. Clarify Rules and Responsibilities

It's not uncommon to hear practice owners and managers complain about employees arguing over who should be doing what responsibilities and how these tasks should be done. It's also not uncommon to hear the same complaints around office rules and policies. For example, employees who disagree on how to handle a patient complaint. The problem is not the policy itself. The problem is a lack of unified clarity on what the policies are.

When employees do not fully understand the rules and responsibilities associated with their positions, confusion is the result. Confusion in the workplace will almost always have a negative impact on efficiency and productivity. It will inevitably lead to a lot of mistakes, jobs being done incorrectly, or jobs not being done at all. When rules and responsibilities are not clarified by leadership, it's often the most vocal member of your team who steps up and attempts to tell others how things should be done. This is what happens when there is a leadership void in an organization.

Proper clarification is the antidote for unnecessary confusion. It leads to streamlined operations, improved employee satisfaction and better business outcomes.

Follow the steps below:

1. Establish your rules. All office rules and policies need to be understandable and clear. If you don't have an employee manual, then work with a professional to have one created. This should include regulations, policies and consequences that apply in any workplace situation. Some examples include tardiness, dress code and etiquette.

2. Create job descriptions. This can change over time as new employees are hired with different strengths and attributes (the focus of week 4), but it's important that each employee is clear on their responsibilities and expectations. This will also assist you when hiring new employees, as both sides will be clear on what the job duties entail.

3. Establish a chain of command. In small business, having too many cooks in the kitchen can be counter-productive, and also exasperate further confusion. In some practices, all employees report to the doctor/owner. As a practice gets bigger, many practices promote or hire an office manager. Some offices have multiple managers. It's important that authority and the chain of command is established and clarified. This isn't to suggest a micromanaged, draconian work

environment (more on that in week 2), but employees do need to be clear on who they answer to.

As a side note, go beyond technical skills when clarifying expectations. Patients expect your employees to know *how* to do their job. It's the manner in which they do it that people will remember. Behaviors like smiling, greeting patients when they walk in, and being supportive when other employees need help should be job duties, not requests. Make sure this is written down and reviewed frequently.

There are a few additional things we want to consider when assigning duties and clarifying job descriptions. We'll come back to that in the coming weeks, but for now let's consider your own duties and responsibilities. I want you to write down 3 things you can accomplish this week that will contribute to the goals of the practice. Consider what activities, if done with excellence, will have the greatest impact on getting you closer to the vision you described in part 1. Make this list a priority, not something you will get to if you "have time." Block out time on your schedule if necessary. We all have the same 24 hours in a day. Often times the difference between high and low performers is that high performers prioritize their goals and schedule time in their day to do the important tasks necessary to put them closer to their goals. Even if these individual weekly tasks are small, it's amazing how doing a lot of the small but right things consistently and diligently can lead to massive changes and improvements over time. This applies to both your professional and personal life! Create a new list every week and remember – you have a "team" that can help you! Effective leadership involves delegation.

3. Clarify Why

Ask yourself, why does our practice exist? Are you in the "glasses and contact lens" business, or are you in the "service" business? As in, we exist to *serve* people by improving their lives through better vision? As a business serving your community, what is your mission? If you don't have one, give this some thought and write one down. Once you have a written mission statement, communicate this to the staff. There are thousands of items that could end up on the to-do list of a business owner, but clarity around a vision and mission helps narrow down that to-do list. Focus and prioritization are of utmost importance to reaching goals!

Research shows that compared with ineffective leaders, high performing leaders have more clarity on who they are, what they want, how to get it, and what they find meaningful and fulfilling. As mentioned above, they are also adept at communicating this vision to others. If you can increase someone's clarity, you will likely up their performance as well. Leadership starts with clarity!

Featured Resources:

Want to learn how great leaders inspire action? Check out this Ted Talk by Simon Sinek. https://bit.ly/2DYKkXY Think about this when you're creating your "Why" story above. Is there a greater purpose to what you do than just sell eyewear? Can you rally your staff around this purpose?

You've written down your vision and goals, but maybe you're still not convinced you'll have time for doing the "extra things" necessary to achieve your goals? Kids, deadlines, putting out fires, etc.!! Watch this video by Stephen Covey, author of *7 Habits of Highly Effective People*. https://bit.ly/2fAGZpU Maybe the problem is not lack of time, but rather lack of prioritization?

A Word on Culture:

It's important that your staff understands the broader goals and vision of the practice, what is expected of them in terms of rules and responsibilities, and "why" it's important for everyone to contribute. But as you can probably guess, performing this simple exercise once and giving it very limited attention afterward is not likely to deliver lasting change. Office culture takes time to develop and takes time to change. Continually and diligently providing clarity for your team around these areas is necessary to cause lasting impact on office culture. The goal is not perfection; the goal is steady and continuous improvement. For most small to mid-sized businesses with limited time and resources, steady often wins the race.

I also want to be clear that I do not think there is one *right* leadership style. The workplace is too complex to distill leadership down to a simple formula. Throughout this course, I openly invite you to ask questions as well as challenge my assertions. I admit I'm somewhat biased by what I've seen work, but I'm open to new ideas and findings that lead us down the path of better understanding humans and how they work. Along the way, I'd love to hear what works for you and what doesn't. Within each lesson remains room for flexibility. Surely there will be many things mentioned that you are already doing, but I encourage you to apply new ideas to your workplace and do your own research. Test new ideas and observe the results over time. I merely suggest you keep doing what works for you and discard the rest. Becoming an effective leader has much less to do with innate leadership skills as it does developing deliberate habits that you execute on a routine basis.

What's Next?

One of the goals of this course is to make your job as owner or manager easier, not harder. If you're of the mindset that you constantly need to be managing (sometimes micro-managing) people to get results, you will likely fall short of being an effective leader. In fact, the *need* to constantly micromanage people is often the byproduct of failed leadership. I want you to be surrounded by a team that isn't entirely dependent on you and can think and act for themselves. It starts with providing clarity, but it certainly doesn't end there. That's the focus of next week's lesson.

Week 2: Empower Your Team

Welcome to week 2 of Eye on Leadership, a 5-week course designed to make you a better leader!

In this course, you can expect to get:

- A vision of what it means to be a great leader
- A powerful framework for solving staff management problems
- Practical leadership skills you can begin using tomorrow
- A specific process and action-plan to get you started

In short, you will get the mind-set, skill-set and tool-set necessary to create a motivated and engaged team and achieve your goals.

Lesson 2: Empower Your Team

In week 1, we discussed setting clear expectations for employees. Failure to provide clarity around goals and expectations for employees is often a leader's first failure. If people do not know *what* is expected of them; how can they be expected to succeed?

However, nowhere in lesson 1 did I suggest micromanaging people or dictating their jobs to them. Having authority might make you a "boss" of others, but it doesn't necessarily mean you will be an effective leader or manager. There is a term called positional leadership. These are leaders who are in charge solely on the basis of their position or title. Considering the #1 reason people leave jobs is because of a negative relationship with a boss or supervisor, it's clear to see how hierarchy alone does not qualify one as an effective leader.

Listening to your employees and valuing their input does not mean that you, as a leader, do not have control and authority over other employees. In fact, it's important that authority is established for those in managerial and leadership positions. People need to be clear on *who* is in charge. However; many great leaders are credited with having a certain level of humility. In fact, having personally worked with numerous practice managers from all sizes of practices, I can tell you that almost without exception the most successful managers had one trait in common. Each one cared more about the practice than their title. It wasn't about having authority or imposing their will on others; rather it was rallying their team around common goals. Humility involves a willingness to involve others and listen to their ideas. Ego and humility cannot coexist. The best leaders and managers I've worked with had much more of the latter than the former.

Week 2 Assignments:

1. Read chapter 3 of *Eye on Leadership* – The Smartest Guy in the Room

2. Ask each employee to complete a Staff Self-Assessment Survey (see example below). Upon completion of this course, I'm going to ask you to start having quarterly (more frequent if necessary) one-on-one meetings with each employee. Ask employees to complete this prior to their first meeting with you.

3. If you're not already having staff meetings, start having these weekly. Staff meetings can be extremely valuable and a great forum for providing the clarity we discussed in Chapter 1. Many of the challenges I hear from practice owners and managers would benefit from the collective brainstorming of the team. Make a list of 1- 3 problems or challenges your office

is facing and invite employees to offer their input, ideas and solutions. To avoid these meetings becoming gripe sessions, set one very important guideline – if you're going to bring a problem, you have to also bring a proposed solution.

---

7 Ways To Empower Employees (Without Losing Control)

Establish guardrails. Employees should be permitted to make some of their own decisions, but there needs to be clarity on the boundaries. Micromanagement restricts employees. Boundaries empower them. A good example would be allowing your employees to use up to $200 to resolve a patient complaint on the spot without consulting a manager.

Listen intently. Not listening to your employee's ideas is a surefire way to get them to stop coming to you with ideas. One of the biggest drawbacks to an organization that doesn't listen to its employees is that commitment and motivation wane, while you lose out on potentially valuable insight from the people you hire.

Lean into people's strengths. One of the reasons some managers struggle to relinquish control is because they fear the employee will not do the job right. Another approach is to lean into people's strengths and give them the freedom to do more of what they are good at. Maybe even *better* than you!

Forgive mistakes. Allowing your employees some autonomy to do their jobs without continuous oversight will not come without some bumps in the road. Punishing every mistake will lead to a staff that fears independence and struggles to make decisions on their own. If you were clear on the guardrails mentioned above, then most of these mistakes should be acceptable learning experiences vs. mission critical offenses.

Ask questions vs. dictate answers. Questions can be very powerful and also communicate to the recipient that you value their input. For example, "How can we increase our capture rate in the optical?" You may already have ideas on how to accomplish this, but you may also hear fresh ideas you had not considered. People like to see their own ideas succeed, so instead of dictating answers to people that reflect one person's opinion (yours), invite your team to get involved as well and see if they bring a higher level of energy into making it a success.

Get a commitment. There is a psychological component to this one. Studies have found that once someone makes a public commitment to another person to do something, that person feels a larger sense of obligation to act in accordance with their commitment. For ex., "I need you to reduce our accounts receivable by 30% by the end of the month. Can you do that for me?" Once they answer yes, they have made a commitment to you. This may not *always* work, but it beats having to continuously badger someone to do their job.

Earn people's trust. It's not enough to just say you empower your employees, they have to believe you. If you can't help yourself from constantly micromanaging your employees and reprimanding every decision that doesn't align with your exact preference, then employees will not truly feel empowered.

Don't Lose Focus!

I would like you to review the vision you clarified in Lesson 1. Keep this written vision statement somewhere it will be regularly seen. Research has shown that regularly monitoring your goals is just as important to the attainment of the goal as setting the goal in the first place. If you're feeling ambitious, I suggest you create a weekly or even daily habit of writing down this vision on a fresh sheet of paper to reinforce the image in your mind. Bring more detail and "feeling" to this vision each time. I want this vision engrained in your memory and a driving force in your business decisions. Clarity can quickly fade as we get caught up in the daily grind of operating a business and our personal lives as well. We become more reactive to problems and less proactive to executing strategic change. Before we know it, our goals and dreams become nothing more than unrealized ideas jotted down on a piece of paper and stuffed into a drawer. For a leader, it's important that clarity is maintained and all activities, including those of your employees, are mapped to the achievement of these goals. Don't lose focus!

Featured Resources:

In this short video, Steve Jobs talks about managing people. Near the end of the video, listen to what he says after "If you want to hire great people and have them stay working for you…" Video: https://bit.ly/1khGb1W

Bonus video: Watch Jim Collins, author of *Good to Great: Why Some Companies Make the Leap.. And Others Don't*, discussing the KEY ATTRIBUTE of the great leaders he studied. Video: https://bit.ly/1khGb1W

What's Next?

Admittedly, lesson 2 and 3 should probably be reversed. I say that because before you can comfortably allow for some level of autonomy and independence in the workplace that allows employees to feel empowered, it's a leader's responsibility to 'clear the path' for them to succeed without constant oversight and supervision. Clearing the path involves providing clarity around expectations, goals and priorities, but clarity is only half the equation. Next week we'll discuss the other half. Clarity covers the "what", but not the "how". If you're giving responsibilities to your employees without providing support for them in both of these areas, you are not empowering them – you are abandoning them!

INSERT PRACTICE NAME

Employee Survey

We would like your participation in an employee survey to learn more about how you feel about your employment with (Insert Company Name), and how we can improve as an employer. All answers will remain confidential between you and your manager. We appreciate your honest and open communication.

Your Name:

1. List 3 things you enjoy about your job.

_____

_____

_____

2. What do you see as your major strength(s)?

_____

_____

_____

3. Do you feel Management recognizes your abilities?

☐ Yes, Occasionally

☐ Often

☐ Not At All

4. Name one thing you believe you could work on and improve?

_____

_____

_____

5. How can Management help you accomplish this?

_____

_____

_____

6. How often do you meet with your Supervisor to discuss your work?

_____

_____

_____

7. List 3 things you would like further training on.

8. What position other than your current one, if any, would you like to have?

9. Who are your favorite staff members to work with?

10. Have you noticed any staff conflict that is unresolved?

    ☐ Yes, if yes, please describe below.

    ☐ No

11. How can the Practice as a whole improve patient care?

_____

_____

_____

12. Do you feel you are compensated fairly for the work that you do?

☐ Yes

☐ No

13. Why or Why Not?

_____

_____

_____

14. Other than cash compensation, what benefit would make you happier at work?

_____

_____

_____

Week 3: Employee Training & Development

Welcome to week 3 of Eye on Leadership, a 5-week course designed to make you a better leader!

In this course, you can expect to get:

- A vision of what it means to be a great leader
- A powerful framework for solving staff management problems
- Practical leadership skills you can begin using tomorrow
- A specific process and action-plan to get you started

In short, you will get the mind-set, skill-set and tool-set necessary to create a motivated and engaged team and achieve your goals.

Lesson 3: Employee Training & Development

In week 1 we focused on clarity. In week 2 we discussed empowering employees. Both are critical components to having a team that can successfully operate without continuous supervision and oversight. But one key ingredient is missing – training and development!

Here are a few questions I commonly hear from consulting members. Isn't there a website I can direct my staff to for training? Is there a class I can send them to? Will you come and train my staff?

Employee training… this seems to be something nobody wants to do. To answer the above questions, yes, there are outside resources available for training staff. However; it's best to utilize these resources as a supplement to your internal training process, not a replacement. In a service industry, employee training and development are too important to completely delegate. After all, nobody knows your culture and brand better than you. Why would you completely delegate this responsibility to a 3rd party?

But we don't have time! Yes, I understand there is limited time for many owners and managers, but as I try to stress in the book, investing more time on the front end with staff training often leads to less work on the back end. Too often the approach to training staff is very haphazard and inconsistent. New hires are trained by current employees often unqualified to do training. Poor techniques and bad habits get passed down. Important aspects of training get overlooked. There is no "system" for training and the results are often predictable. There remains a lack of certainty around how to do various tasks, numerous mistakes are made, and management ends up spending excessive time managing the wrong things – like fixing all the mistakes that occur from poor training! Where staff training is lacking, managers end up spending more time managing employees, not less.

For tips on training new hires, see section below: How to Train New Employees

---

Week 3 Assignments:

1. Read chapter 4 of Eye on Leadership – Coach Kevin

2. Create a Training Manual for new hires that includes steps and procedures for job tasks. This can also serve as a guide that employees can refer back to. This should include objectives and deadlines for new hires, with reasonable flexibilities described below. Be patient and understand at times you will have to re-train. To ensure competence, require the trainee to demonstrate a task, not just acknowledge that he or she understands.

A good time to create a Training Manual for new hires is during training. As you're training a new hire, document the steps involved in performing job duties and use this to create a training manual. Allowing employees to train new hires as they see fit allows too much room for human error and inconsistencies. Having a training "system" that's supervised by a manager or experienced employee is preferable and ensures new hires are adequately trained in all aspects of their job description.

Employee Development

Maybe it's just a matter of semantics, but I don't consider training and development the same thing. I consider training the process of giving somebody the rudimentary skills they need to do a job. For many employers this is where it ends. But for other employers, this is only the beginning. Employee development is an investment in the *continuous* growth and development of the employee. The result is the character Sam in the book, as opposed to the disengaged employee who only serves to perform routine tasks and process transactions. To get a high-performing, motivated team, employees must continually be developed. We'll revisit this in Lesson 5, but for now give some thought to additional ways you could continue to invest in your employees – classes, seminars, presentation from reps, etc.

Consider both technical competence and service aspects of employee development. How close to "mastery" can you get your employees? See the video below.

Featured Resource:

Daniel Pink, author of *Drive: The surprising truth about what motivates us*, uncovered some interesting insight on 3 factors that lead to better performance. The science, as he describes it, is a little "freaky". Video: https://bit.ly/1gNxOdQ

What's Next?

It is possible for employees to be clear on what is expected of them, be adequately trained and be given a reasonable amount of autonomy in their role, yet still fail to perform at a level they are capable of. Next week we'll explore a common reason, and how to address it.

How To Train New Employees

Finally, help is on the way! The new hire will begin training tomorrow... Properly training newly hired employees is essential to companies and their employees. Failure to provide adequate training results in job dissatisfaction that leads to high rates of staff turnover.

Many practices are already stretched thin with personnel. Even with adequate personnel, your staff may be very busy with current job responsibilities. Nevertheless, adequately training new hires has become a dirty job that someone has to do, but who? And how?

Step 1: Delegate training responsibilities wisely.

Unfortunately, the job of training is often assigned to those within the closest proximity to the new hire and to those with the most available time. It's imperative that the individual(s) providing the training have the necessary skills to be effective. Educating the trainer(s) is an important first step in successfully training new hires.

Step 2: Socially and professionally mentor the new hire.

A friendly, knowledgeable and positive co-worker can be a valuable resource person for the trainee, bridging gaps that all newly hired individual's experience.

Step 3: Put it in writing.

Provide or create a written training manual that contains specific instructions and reference information. It will be a valuable resource for the new employee and will hasten his/her success.

Step 4: Create a safe learning environment.

It's the trainer's responsibility to create a non-threatening environment for learning. The most effective way to achieve that is to establish a relationship with the trainee. People skills are vital to establishing a relaxed and friendly learning environment. Take the time to engage in conversation with the newcomer, asking about his/her family, hobbies and interests, and don't forget to share your own. Professional business settings are comprised of human beings, so act like one...and treat the newly hired person as you would like to be treated.

Step 5: Make allowances.

Allow the newly hired employee some latitude in setting the pace of learning new tasks, particularly when the training is provided by numerous employees who must perform their duties as well as train the new hire. In a busy, hectic environment, that is a huge challenge for all to overcome.

Step 6: Provide the tools to succeed.

Present the newly hired employee with a notebook that includes a comprehensive job description. It's a valuable assessment tool. Measuring progress based upon the job description builds the newly hired employee's confidence through affirmation of the trainee's accomplishments.

Step 7: Eliminate roadblocks.

Negativity is a roadblock to learning. Praise and positive feedback reinforce and affirm the efforts of everyone. Expect and provide positive interactions and feedback. There are no training shortcuts, therefore, allow time and repetition to bring the results everyone wants. Avoid the temptation to dictate and micro-manage the learning timeframe. Setting and expressing unreasonable timeframe goals are among the biggest roadblocks to the new hire success.

Step 8: Segment the training. As the trainee acquires the knowledge and skills to perform a complex task well, he/she will also gain confidence. Confidence is an empowering catalyst that enables the trainee to move on to mastering the next segment, accelerating the process.

Step 9: Shelve cross-training ideals. Put cross training on the shelf until the trainee has accomplished a measure of success performing the duties outlined on his/her job description. Spare the trainee from the added stress of learning two roles until they are competent in their primary role.

Step 10: Be generous with praise, stingy with criticism.

Grandma taught us that we catch more flies with honey than with vinegar. Keep that thought in mind when dealing with a new employee's errors. Coming down hard on a new employee who's attempting to learn what it's taken the rest of the staff months and years to learn impedes learning. It's counter-productive.

Step 11: Don't micro-manage.

Micro-management is the biggest deterrent there is to learning and productivity. Micro-managing employees sends the signal of a lack of confidence in the trainee's capabilities. Micro-managing sends many trainees out the door!

Step 12: Final tips.

Every business has its share of hurdles to overcome, including training and retaining newly hired employees. In business, time and money are one and the same, and it takes both to train a new employee. Any company or organization that laments its high rate of new-staff turnover needs to re-evaluate how newly hired staff is trained to determine whether inadequate training may indeed be the culprit.

Week 4: Discover Your (Employee's) Strengths

Welcome to week 4 of Eye on Leadership, a 5-week course designed to make you a better leader!

In this course, you can expect to get:

- A vision of what it means to be a great leader
- A powerful framework for solving staff management problems
- Practical leadership skills you can begin using tomorrow
- A specific process and action-plan to get you started

In short, you will get the mind-set, skill-set and tool-set necessary to create a motivated and engaged team and achieve your goals.

Lesson 4: Discover Your (Employee's) Strengths

How do I fix my employees? Maybe not in those exact words, but that's the essence of the question I often hear directed at underperforming employees. How can I fix these real or perceived weaknesses that are preventing them from doing their best work?

The reality, we *all* have strengths and we all have weaknesses. Certainly, some of our weaknesses would benefit from additional coaching or training, but we all have certain character flaws that can be very resistant to change. Someone who is very shy and introverted may never shine in a sales role. An employee who lacks attention to detail may not be the best fit as your billing person. Someone who lacks empathy and patience may find a management role challenging. It's much more difficult, if not impossible, to train these hard-wired qualities. In term of getting the best work out of employees, would it be more effective to align employee's job duties and responsibilities with their strengths?

Fix Weaknesses or Double Down On Strengths?

Each person's greatest value to the organization and potential for growth is found in their strengths. Whether it's work, home or in the community, people are more likely to reach their maximum potential when they get to use their true talents. In most cases, there is also a correlation between people's strengths and their level of enjoyment when their job responsibilities are aligned with their strengths. While I'm sure there are exceptions, I don't know too many great athletes who don't like sports. We typically bring a higher level of energy to things that are interesting to us, especially when we are good at that activity. If you're a parent, you've probably exposed your child at a young age to many different activities, but eventually the child gravitates toward activities that he or she is talented at and enjoys doing. Most parents will support and nurture the child's pursuit of these activities. These are the activities the child is more likely to excel at.

Week 3 focused on employee training and development. If you want your team to consistently perform at a high level that earns high praise (and referrals) from patients, you have to be constantly investing in their growth. That said, be careful not to overlook people's natural strengths. Sometimes managers take natural talents for granted and focus all their time trying to fix people's weaknesses. If you are always in "self-improvement" mode, you can expect an uphill battle.

2 incorrect assumptions:

- Employees can become competent at anything if they are trained properly.

- An employee's greatest potential for growth is found in improving or minimizing his or her weaknesses.

Instead:

- Many of our strengths and weaknesses are hard-wired. For example, even with extensive management training, someone with poor communication skills will likely struggle to succeed in a leadership role.

- Each person's greatest areas of opportunity and growth are found in their strengths. People can improve in their job by working on their weaknesses, but if the goal is to have more employees who "excel" in their role, allow them to maximize their strengths.

Fatal weaknesses

Ask yourself if the weakness is too insurmountable to allow the employee to continue to work in your practice. For example, an employee who has an abrasive personality that is disrupting teamwork and morale in the office. If you've discussed this with the employee and it continues to be a problem, then you may have to cut ties with this individual. But also consider if a weakness is something that can be managed around. This is where flexibility in job responsibilities comes into play. I've talked a few owner ODs out of terminating a high-performing employee who struggled in one or two non-critical areas. "But everyone needs to know how to do this, and he keeps messing up!" In the end, we agreed that some flexibility in job responsibilities was preferable to losing a valuable employee.

One of a manager's greatest frustrations is providing a lot of training and coaching and the employee continues to under-perform. Developing your employee's knowledge (facts) and skills (the steps of an activity) is wise, but it won't overcome a lack of talent. I'll pick on doctors here. We gain a lot of knowledge in optometry school. We learn how to competently perform a lot of tests. While this makes us good doctors from a clinical standpoint, it won't overcome a lack of talent in areas like empathy and chairside manner. If you are hiring an associate OD, would it be better to hire for these strengths, or spend a lot of time trying to fix these weaknesses?

The truth about strengths is that to most of us, they don't even feel like strengths. These are the thoughts, feeling and behaviors that just feel natural to us. This is why it's hard to fix weaknesses in areas where strengths are lacking. In many cases, you're asking someone to consistently perform and behave in ways that do not feel natural to them.

Week 4 Assignments:

1. Read chapter 5 of Eye on Leadership – The Self-Improvement Fallacy

2. Based on your observations, write down 1 - 3 strengths and 1 - 3 weaknesses for each employee.

3. Compare your list with the information provided by the employee on the Staff Self-Assessment Survey you asked the employees to complete in week 2. This information will be applied when you discuss roles and responsibilities with employees in your upcoming one-on-ones. For now, take a preliminary assessment on whether everyone's job responsibilities are aligned with their strengths and areas of interest. Are you maximizing the talent in your practice, or wasting it?

Featured Resource:

In this lesson, we mostly focus on evaluating the strengths and weaknesses of your employees. It would be a huge oversight to not also evaluate your own strengths and weaknesses as a leader. There are a lot of good books and resources available to help people assess their individual strengths. Certainly not the only option, but I'll mention a book I read several years ago that I found very helpful in my own personal development. The book is called *Now, Discover Your Strengths* and you can find it here: https://amzn.to/2GJoo6U

I would also recommend offering Personality Assessment Tests to your employees. We offer these tests for consulting members. These are very beneficial for hiring purposes and also evaluating if employees are positioned in the appropriate roles. Two of the most popular tests are The Myer-Briggs Type Indicator and the DISC assessment. Another test we used at IDOC was based on the book *Personality Plus* by Florence Littauer. https://amzn.to/2tBgzYa

---

What's Next?

As discussed in week 1, communication is critical to becoming an effective leader. It's time to meet with your team and make sure everyone is on the same page. Next week we'll bring everything together and create a plan for continued growth and improvement – led by you!

Week 5: Accountability

Welcome to week 5 of Eye on Leadership, a 5-week course designed to make you a better leader!

In this course, you can expect to get:

- A vision of what it means to be a great leader
- A powerful framework for solving staff management problems
- Practical leadership skills you can begin using tomorrow
- A specific process and action-plan to get you started

In short, you will get the mind-set, skill-set and tool-set necessary to create a motivated and engaged team and achieve your goals.

Lesson 5: Accountability

Congratulation! You've reached the final week of the Eye on Leadership training course. Hopefully you've following along with the lessons and assignments. I saved this lesson for last, because accountability is the glue that holds it all together. Without holding team members accountable for outcomes, it's unlikely you will see lasting change. The "clear" vision you wrote down in lesson one will start to become increasingly blurry and out of reach as efforts at change and improvement will be displaced by the unwelcome return of the status quo. "We tried it for a while, but the staff went back to doing things the old way."

How do I hold people accountable?

There are a lot of misconceptions around accountability. It conjures up images of people in positions of authority constantly looking over the shoulder of others to make sure they are doing their job correctly and reprimanding them when they fail. I think we all know the word for that type of leadership – it's micromanagement! I hope by now you realize the reasons micromanagement has its drawbacks. Not to mention, the need to micromanage employees is often a result of failure to provide adequate clarity, coaching and support necessary for employees to succeed without constant supervision.

Perhaps the biggest excuse I hear for not holding employees accountable is "I don't like confrontation." I don't like confrontation either. Most people don't. Sometimes confrontation is unavoidable, but I prefer a process that effectively holds employees accountable WITHOUT the need for awkward confrontation.

Accountability is synonymous with "answerability." It's simply a process of getting employees to perform in a way in which they know in advance they will have to regularly "account" for their performance. This requires a lot of communication! As you'll read in the final chapters of the book, one of the most effective things you can do in terms of managing staff is meet regularly with each employee in a one-on-one setting. Too often these one-on-one meetings only occur when there's a problem. If you want to avoid many of these problems, the antidote is more frequent and high-level communication.

This is the part where I recommend setting up regular one-on-one meetings with each employee. These meetings do not need to be lengthy or formal. Nor are they intended to reprimand poor performers without first understanding all the facts. Enter these meetings with 3 objectives in mind. It's an opportunity to touch base with the employee and learn of any problems or challenges they are facing in their role. It's an opportunity to recognize the employee's positive attributes and contributions. In addition to making the employee feel valued, this is also information the employee needs to continue succeeding in his or her role. People tend to want to repeat behaviors that earn them praise. Lastly, it's an opportunity to address areas of underperformance. The final chapter of the book goes into more detail on this.

The assignments below tie everything together that we've discussed.

Week 5 Assignments:

1. Read chapter 6 (The Setback) and the Conclusion of Eye on Leadership

2. Schedule one-on-one meetings with each employee.

   a. Review Job duties. Ensure alignment and understanding with job duties and expectations. Before finalizing job duties, review the survey you asked each employee to complete in Week 2. Consider the strengths and interests of the employee. Are the employee's duties and responsibilities aligned with his or her strengths and interests? Is everyone in the right seat on the bus?

   b. Complete a 90-Day Evaluation Form (sample below). Involve the employee in setting goals and action plans.

c. Create an employee development plan. What aspects of the job does the employee want or need more help with? What would you like him or her to learn or become more skilled at? This may require further training by management, outside assistance like a training course or demo from a rep, or an agreement that the employee will use their down time for self-study.

d. Schedule your next meeting where the initiatives above will be revisited, and the employee will be asked to report on progress and outcomes.

Accountability

Accountability will be reinforced in these follow-up one-on-one meetings. I don't want to overlook staff meetings as well. Staff meetings also provide a forum to review performance and expectations and hold the team accountable for results, but staff meetings have their limitations. As discussed in the book, low performers can sometimes hide out at staff meetings without having to account for their individual performance. And quite frankly, a staff meeting is not the appropriate forum for addressing poor performance by individual employees. Nonetheless, keep having staff and/or departmental meetings, but work in one-on-one meetings also. When employees know they can no longer continue to underperform without fear of having to answer for their poor performance, accountability will be established.

What if they are not improving?

That's a possibility. But I suggest you first give the employee the benefit of the doubt. Seek to learn more about the situation. Get curious! Sometimes employees have valid reasons for not performing at the expected level. Maybe their workload is too great and they are struggling to complete all their tasks. Maybe they need more training to perform a certain task without making so many errors. Under these scenarios, management steps in to provide the necessary support and training. However, sometimes the problem is not under-management; the problem is the employee. Employees who are not coachable, resistant to change, or noncompliant are difficult to fix – even in an environment where supportive management exists. When that's the case, you essentially have 3 choices:

1. Can we live with the employee's shortcomings?

2. Can we move the employee to another position that better suits his or her strengths and competencies?

3. Would we be better off parting ways?

In closing, one of the most common challenges I hear from practice owners and managers involves managing staff. It's unusual for a practice to not have at least one or two underperformers on the team. Some examples are more extreme than others. Nonetheless, when an owner or manager is singling out an underperformer, my initial objective as a consultant is to determine if this is an employee problem or a management problem. Interestingly, a "bad hire" and a poorly managed employee look very similar in terms of their workplace performance. Both are likely to struggle in their role. My goal for this course was to give you the tools to increase the performance and production of those employees willing to contribute at a higher level. If you execute on the ideas taught in this course, you can have better assurance that you've done your part as a leader – perhaps making the 3rd option above justified.

I hope you found this 5-week course helpful. If you were already doing a lot of these things, then great! Rest assured you were on the right path. And if it hasn't occurred to you yet, leadership is not only important in the workplace, it's important in life! Here's to your success!

I would love to hear your thoughts on this course! Please email them to me at Svargo@idoc.net.

90 Day Evaluation Form

Performance Rating Scale

1. ***Does Not Meet Expectations:*** Sometimes meets performance expectations but often falls short of expectations; requires repeated guidance and supervision in executing normal expectations. Inconsistent demonstration of necessary skills for the position; improved performance is required.

2. ***Meets Expectation:*** Always achieves and occasionally exceeds performance objectives while demonstrating required behaviors and values; is recognized as a solid contributor to the organization and the team; executes goals and responsibilities with some guidance; when directed, significantly contributes to the achievement of individual and organizational goals and objectives.

3. ***Exceeds Expectation:*** Consistently exceeds expected performance results while always exhibiting desired behaviors and values; executes goals and responsibilities with minimal guidance; demonstrates strong expertise in relevant skills and seeks new knowledge and skills to meet future organizational challenges; is proactive in planning and organizing for future organizational growth needs.

Performance Expectation	(1)	(2)	(3)
Job Knowledge: Fully understands job responsibilities, procedures, scope of duties, and work methods.			
Productivity: Produces the quality and volume of work one might reasonably expect and accepts accountability for the work product.			
Service Quality: Effectively participates as a member of the team in identifying and improving work processes to better serve our members.			
Job Results: Is accountable for results and actions; tracks activities and provides follow-up as necessary; assures tasks are completed on time.			
Interactions with Others: Develops and maintains an effective working relationship with others at various levels inside and outside the organization.			
Commitment to Work: Demonstrates a consistent and reliable work effort; applies a sense of urgency to complete tasks in order to meet service expectations, whether planned or unplanned.			

Step 1. Improvement Goals: These are the goals related to areas of concern to be improved:

1.

2.

3.

Step 2. Activity Goals: Listed are the activities that will help you reach your goals:

1.

2.

3.

4.

5.

Step 3. Progress Checkpoints: The following schedule will be used to evaluate your progress in meeting your improvement activities.

Goal 1- Checkpoint Date:

Progress Expected:

Progress Made:

Goal 2- Checkpoint Date:

Progress Expected:

Progress Made:

Goal 3- Checkpoint Date:

Progress Expected:

Progress Made:

About the Author

Steve Vargo, OD, MBA is a 1998 graduate of the Illinois College of Optometry. In 2014 he joined Prima Eye Group (now IDOC) as Vice President of Optometric Consulting. A published author and speaker with 15 years of clinical experience, he now serves as IDOC's Optometric Practice Management Consultant. Since transitioning to a full-time practice management consultant, Dr. Vargo has performed over 3,000 consultations and coaching sessions with hundreds of independent optometry practices across the country. He speaks regularly at industry conferences, has been published in numerous industry publications, has a regular column in Optometric Management titled "The CEO Checklist", and is a contributing author to the widely read "Optometric Management Tip of the Week" article. Dr. Vargo has authored 3 books on the subjects of staff management, leadership and selling.

Dr. Vargo's other books
(both available on Amazon):

Eye on Management: Step-by-step guide to optometry's most common staff management challenges

But I Don't Sell: An eye care professional's guide to being more persuasive, influential and successful

Questions or Comments?

I'd love to hear your thoughts. Email me at: Svargo@idoc.net.

NEED HELP?

I offer consulting services to independent eye care practices through IDOC. I'll help you transform your staff and your practice. Learn more at www.IDOC.net.

Made in the USA
Middletown, DE
28 March 2022

63281046R00097